CW01508656

March of the Matrons

Military Influence on the British Civilian Nursing Profession, 1939-1969

Penny Starns

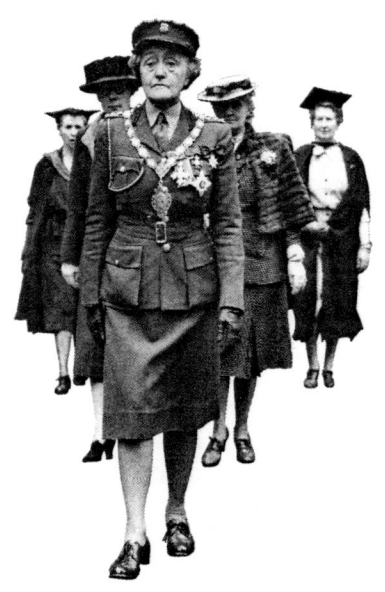

dsm

First published 2000
by DSM
The Studio
Denton
Peterborough
Cambs PE7 3SD

All Rights Reserved.
No part of this publication may be reproduced, stored in a retrieval system, or transmitted, in any form or by any means, electronic, mechanical, photocopying, recording or otherwise without prior permission, in writing, of the publishers and copyright holder.

A catalogue record of this book is available from the British Library.

ISBN 0953651622

Copyright © 2000 Penny Starns

Designed and produced by
DSM
The Studio
Denton
Peterborough
Cambs PE7 3SD

Cover design by Marc Lowen

This book is dedicated
with love to the memory of
Eric John Butler (1950-1973)

Acknowledgements

The research for this book was originally conducted for my PhD thesis and I would like to take this opportunity to thank the University of Bristol and the Power-Postan Foundation of the Economic History Society London School of Economics for funding this research.

I am greatly indebted to my supervisor Professor Rodney Lowe, and to Phil Ollerenshaw, Bob Moore and Anne Marie Rafferty for their critical comments and advice. The research process was greatly assisted by many efficient and helpful archivists, in particular Elizabeth Boardman, Jonathan Evans, Susan McGann and Major McCombe. The kind co-operation of Brian Salmon CBE and Colonel Gruber von Arni RRC was extremely valuable, and special thanks are due to Professor Roger Cooter, Dr Mark Harrison and the late Dr Monica Baly for their constant encouragement and support.

My heartfelt appreciation also goes out to my friends and family, Jo Denman, Charlotte Hooper, Liz Goulding, Ann Starr, Steph Westlake Giorgos Mavros, Joan, Eddie, Lynda and Christopher Starns for listening endlessly to my ideas and arguments and giving me feedback on my work.

Finally I'd like to thank my sons James, Michael and Lewis for their love, humour and patience.

Penny Starns
Bristol 2000

Picture Credits

Royal College of Nursing Archive: *Cover photograph, p195.*

Popperfoto: *Pages 23, 50, 70, 96, 115, 220.*

Contents

List of Abbreviations

Chapter 1
Introduction

Chapter 2
Fighting Militarism? British Nursing during the Second World War

Chapter 3
Revolution or Evolution? The Issue of Nursing Reform

Chapter 4
Changing the Pattern

Chapter 5
Reasserting the Officer

Chapter 6
Masters of their Profession or Slaves to the System?
Nurse Leadership and Nursing Practice

Chapter 7
Uniform Attraction

Chapter 8
Breaking the Mould

Chapter 9
Obedience versus Initiative : The Issue of Nurse Discipline

Chapter 10
Conclusion

Bibliography

Index

List of Abbreviations

AHM	Association of Hospital Matrons
ANTC	Area Nurse Training Committee
ATS	Auxiliary Territorial Service
CHSC	Central Health Services Council
COHSE	Confederation of Health Service Employees
CNO	Chief Nursing Officer
GNC	General Nursing Council
IWM	Imperial War Museum
MRC	Modern Record Centre Warwick
NHS	National Health Service
NUPE	National Union of Public Employees
PMRAFNS	Princess Mary's Royal Air Force Nursing Service
QAIMNS	Queen Alexandra's Imperial Military Nursing Service, post-war
QARANC	Queen Alexandra's Royal Army Nursing Corps
QARNNS	Queen Alexandra's Royal Naval Nursing Service
RAMC	Royal Army Medical Corps
RCN	Royal College of Nursing
RCNA	Royal College of Nursing Archives
RMN	Registered Mental Nurse
RMPA	Royal Medico-Psychological Association
SEAN	State Enrolled Assistant Nurse
SNAC	Standing Nursing Advisory Committee
SRN	State Registered Nurse
TANS	Territorial Army Nursing Service
VAD	Voluntary Aid Detachment
WHO	World Health Organisation

Foreword
by
Chris Watson,
President, Royal College of Nursing

The late Monica Baly, one of nursing's leading historians, observed that if nurses 'do not know where they have come from they will not know where they are going, and if they do not understand the past, they will be destined for ever to repeat its mistakes'.

Penny Starns' assessment of the military influence on nursing makes a valuable contribution to this process. We gain a fascinating perspective on many of the most pressing issues which continue to preoccupy the profession today. The military dimension provides an insight into our deliberations over nurse education and nursing leadership in particular - not forgetting Matron's role, of course.

From Florence Nightingale's days at Scutari, the links between nursing's story and military life have proved highly significant. Comprehending exactly what this legacy means is important as we enter an era in which nurses are extending their practice and are also determined to remain responsible for the essentials of patient care.

As President of the Royal College of Nursing and a member of the RCN's History of Nursing Society, I congratulate Penny Starns on her achievement in adding to our knowledge of nursing's past and understanding of its present and future.

Chris Watson

Chapter 1

Introduction

In recent years there has been a resurgence of interest in the history of British nursing. Nevertheless, the focus has remained almost exclusively on civilian rather than military nursing. The two experiences of civilian and military nurses have been recorded as separate entities and the links between these experiences largely ignored. *Angels and Citizens* by Anne Summers, which records nursing history in the period leading up to the First World War, represents the only in-depth historical analysis to relate military nursing to civilian society; thus an accepted view of nursing has emerged which maintains that nursing evolved by adopting a series of professionalisation strategies in order to gain credibility and status. This book will challenge the professionalisation model of nursing history by arguing that nurses frequently turned to militarisation rather than professionalisation in an effort to raise and protect their status. It will be argued that the military imposition of an outdated military model on civilian nursing from 1945 onwards was responsible for hindering professional progress and preventing reform.

In assessing the military influence on the British nursing profession between 1939 and 1969, it is important to examine the various forces that influenced all professions during this period. Primarily, these forces encompass the historical roots of the profession, recruitment and training strategies, professional membership and leadership, government policy directives and, to some extent, public opinion and media representation. All professions were influenced by the need to meet the demands of society and to respond accordingly to the changing nature of these demands. The structure of this account is therefore largely dictated by the need to examine these influences in greater depth. Since nursing history is important to the wider understanding of both women's social history and the development of healthcare delivery, this study will contribute to both these research areas. By challenging the orthodox view of nursing history a new perspective is gained, that of a pervading military ethos which ultimately acted as an obstacle to change in all aspects of nursing development.

This introductory chapter will supply an analysis of the existing literature relating to nursing history and discuss the conceptual framework of the book. In addition, since the terms 'militarism' and 'militarisation' are used frequently in the main body of the text, a definition of these terms will be provided. The debates that surround these terms will also be considered. Finally, in order to fully comprehend subsequent analysis, the chapter will include a brief summary of nursing history prior to 1939. Please note that since the contents of this book provide a sequel to previous publications some of the material has been published in 'Medicine War & Modernity'(Sutton 1998) and 'Nurses at War' (Sutton 2000). This material is fundamental to the central debates with regard to the militarisation of nursing, and duplication of this material in the following account is for the benefit of those readers who have not read these previous volumes.

Historiography

Traditional accounts of nursing history have concentrated primarily on the domestic and religious roots of nursing development. While Nightingale reforms have served to dominate nursing history in the 19th century, National Health Service (NHS) reforms have provided a similar focus for the 20th century. The paucity of accounts relating to the inter-war years, and nursing during the Second World War, confirms this preoccupation with Nightingale and the NHS. In addition, scholars have provided overviews of nursing history such as *A History of the Nursing Profession* by Brian Abel-Smith and *A Social Introduction to* Nursing by Dingwall *et al*. However, the time period covered by these studies, which traces nursing history from the 19th century to the present day, leaves little room for an analytical approach. In a similar vein, *Queen Alexandra's Royal Army Nursing Corps* by Juliet Piggott and *One Hundred Years of Army Nursing* by Ian Hay provide overviews of military nursing history. However, with the exception of *Angels and Citizens* by Anne Summers - a study that examines the role of British women as military nurses in the period 1854 to 1914 - links between military and civilian nurses in the 19th and 20th centuries have largely been ignored. As Summers has correctly argued, military nursing history has been 'relegated to a footnote in Nightingale history'.[1]

Clearly then, Nightingale studies do not provide an adequate analysis of military nursing history, nor do they stress the historical links that exist between military and civilian nursing organisations. Instead, these studies concentrate on the domestic and religious aspects of nursing history. While scholars have located the military roots of nursing as being firmly associated with Nightingale reforms, there has been a tendency to assume that this military influence died with Nightingale. Furthermore, although the historiographical preoccupation with Nightingale is reflected in the numerous volumes of literature which document her career and achievements, many of these volumes are not historically accurate. Despite the abundance of literature, the myths that surround the Nightingale legend are only successfully exposed in Dr Baly's analysis entitled *Florence Nightingale and the Nursing Legacy*.

If Nightingale literature sheds little light on the links between military and civilian nursing development, studies of the 20th century NHS reforms have obscured these links completely. In some respects, historians can be forgiven for overlooking the civil-military connection in this later period since Nightingale reforms were almost exclusively concerned with nursing, whereas NHS reforms affected all areas of healthcare delivery. To a large extent, therefore, historiography of post-war nursing has reflected the need to view nurses not in isolation but as an integral part of the healthcare system. However, studies which have concentrated on broad healthcare issues, such as Webster's history of the NHS, have failed to give nurses a suitably high profile, while generalist accounts of nursing history for this period are either too brief to be analytical or not adequately contextualised.

Accounts that provide a more detailed analysis of civilian nursing development are *Behind the Mask* by Christopher Hart and *The Effects of the National Health Service on the Nursing Profession* by Rosemary White. The former concentrates on the relationship between nurses and their unions and the latter on the impact of NHS reforms on nursing organisation. Analytical accounts of military nursing history for the same period simply do not exist. Clearly, however, the practice of systematically excluding military nurses from historical analysis has distorted the overall view of nursing history. Consequently, without exception, historians of post-war nursing have adopted a 'professionalisation' view of nursing development.

Nevertheless, despite the conformity displayed by historians, contemporary studies of the period suggest a different scenario. The measurement of supervisory attitudes undertaken by Professor Revans in 1961, for instance, highlighted the detrimental effects of military influence within the higher echelons of hospital nursing whereas, at the other end of the nursing hierarchy, the stultifying effects of military-style discipline on new recruits was exposed in a study of cadet nursing compiled by Vera Chambers in 1960. In addition, Una Maclean's contemporary sociological analysis of the nursing profession, published in 1974, provided several analogies between nursing and military organisation. Historical studies, by comparison, have alluded to nursing's military roots without exploring the overall impact of military influence on civilian nursing development. The following study therefore aims to rectify this situation.

Conceptual Framework

Historical accounts of a predominantly female profession can be viewed within the context of feminist theory, since it can be argued that the mere existence of a numerically large group of women provided an ideal prerequisite for the development of feminist affiliations. However, the various strands of feminist ideology within the women's movement provided tensions and, occasionally, conflict regarding policy objectives. These tensions centred on whether women possessed specific female qualities that acknowledged 'separateness' but also a legitimate claim to equality with men, or whether women possessed similar qualities to men and were capable of forming a 'humankind' in which gender differences remained irrelevant to equality of citizenship. Radical feminists, therefore, have argued that nursing embodied the traditional nurturing qualities associated with women which allowed nurses to build a power base on essentially female characteristics, whereas liberal feminists have maintained a total aversion to this notion of biological determinism. Moreover, both radical and liberal feminists have expressed diverse attitudes regarding class, ethnicity and race, which have further contributed to the ambiguity of feminist theory.

Similarly, the nursing profession has not fitted neatly into any particular feminist perspective, and nurses did not appear to endorse any clear feminist ideology, although it can be argued that the resistance displayed by female nurses to the introduction of male general nurses was indicative of a belief in biological determinism. It can equally be argued that this resistance was merely designed to protect occupational interests. Moreover, while feminist theory has highlighted the role of patriarchal oppression in the subjugation of women, matriarchal oppression has been ignored, yet nursing history provides ample evidence of the ways in which women have successfully oppressed other women. Therefore, the failure of feminist theory to confront this issue precludes its use as a framework for this study.

Instead, the text adopts a new approach to nursing history and examines the development of nursing from a 'military' perspective. To an extent, the study is based on Shaw's premise, which states that the unprecedented relationship that existed between British military and civilian society during the Second World War produced:

> *... a particular form of warfare-welfare state in which a framework of social democratic reform was conditioned by the centralising, even secretive needs of war mobilisation in 1939-45 and Atlantic defence thereafter.* [2]

It is the evolutionary juncture of Shaw's 'warfare-welfare' state that provides the starting point for this research. However, since analysis frequently refers to 'militarism' and 'militarisation', some explanation of these terms is required.

Within the international debate, the term 'militarism' has frequently been applied to military industrial complexes and the primacy of militaristic foreign policies. It has also referred to the functionality of militarism within the developing socio-economic structures of individual states. However, there is no succinct definition of militarism. Feminist writings during the First World War equated militarism with the use of force, whereby the masculine urge to dominate far outweighed the ability to co-operate in the international arena. These writings were tempered by others who sought to romanticise military ideals and create the heroic soldier figure. Woodrow Wilson stated in 1916 that:

> *Militarism did not consist of any army, or even the existence of a*
> *great army. Militarism is a spirit. It is a point of view.* [3]

Descriptions of militarism during war have differed somewhat from interpretations in peace and, in more recent years, historians have attempted to define militarism in relationship to civil society, both during periods of peace and war.

Gerhard Ritter's work, for instance, has concentrated on the relationship between state politics and military structures,[4] whereas Huntington's analysis has looked more explicitly at military involvement in the socio-economic frameworks of states.[5] These studies have essentially examined the ways in which countries have prepared for war; however, war preparation is not the same as militarism, although arguably one can lead directly to the other. Indeed, militarism is not confined to political and economic spheres but clearly indicates an overriding military influence within civilian society at all levels. According to Berghann, there are two types of militarism. The first type emerged in pre-industrial states and was characterised by:

> *… the self exclusiveness of the military sphere, an emphasis on an*
> *all-pervasive militaristic spirit to be generated by indoctrination*
> *and through paramilitary organisation, and military preparation*
> *by means of an austerity programme.*

The second type surfaced when the industrialisation process incorporated various stages of technology and involved a 'civil military symbiosis'.[6] For clarification purposes, these distinctions are defined as 'aristocratic militarism' and 'technocratic militarism'.

Significantly, historians have assumed that aristocratic militarism gradually succumbed to technocratic militarism with very little overlap in terms of ideology and structure. However, research findings for this study have indicated that it was possible for both forms of militarism to co-exist and that militarisation was directly linked to existing value systems. Furthermore, while militarisation has referred to the growth of militarism, the process occurred at various levels in society at different times, thus it was possible to argue that international diplomacy was militarised and to simultaneously argue that civilian society was demilitarised. However, Shaw's interpretation of militarism and militarisation provides the working definition for this study. Militarism, he argues, 'is not a matter of good or bad, but of how far military organisation and values (which sometimes may be justified and necessary) impinge on social structure',[7] whereas militarisation is the process by which militarism becomes an integral part of civilian society.

Historical and sociological debates in the post-war period have centred on how and why militarisation took place at any given time and whether individual states embarked on demilitarisation programmes. According to Enloe, for example, civil society became increasingly militarised due to the nuclear age, war preparation and insidious civilian participation in military affairs.[8] Conversely, Shaw has claimed that society experienced a demilitarisation process, since war preparation was not necessarily accompanied by militarisation. However, both these statements have referred to a global perspective of militarism and, significantly, Britain did not conform to a global trend. As Shaw has argued, Britain provided 'a strong test case of the survival of militarism in a post-military society'.[9] Post-war conscription was:

> ... *profoundly important to British society. For several generations still alive and active today, National Service - if not actual war experience - became a fundamental experience of the transition to adulthood.* [10]

Furthermore, while Britain was one of the first European states to abandon conscription - an action that suggested the demilitarisation of society - she also harboured military ambitions, which were not shared by her European neighbours. Thus, in terms of military spending, political objectives and existing value systems, British society experienced greater levels of militarism in the 1950s than any other European state. Clearly, therefore, Shaw's view of militarism in Britain converges with that of Enloe. Albeit a paradoxical situation, Britain managed to combine 'structural demilitarisation with continuing cultural, ideological and political forms of militarism'.[11]

Research into British nursing history for this period supports the view that Britain experienced increased levels of militarism from 1939 onwards. However, research has also revealed that between 1950 and 1960 the militarisation process was more intense than during the war years. Specific military values were perceived to be important in the creation of post-war Britain and, since military methods and ambitions were held in high regard, civil society adopted a mixture of military values. Some values were associated with neo-feudalist aristocratic militarism and others with 20th century technocratic militarism. While aristocratic militarism stressed the importance of character and the denigration of intellectual knowledge, 20th century militarism emphasised the virtues of military efficiency and technological progress. By 1945 these two types of militarism were incompatible since advances in technology had exposed the weaknesses of aristocratic militarism. Technology demanded intellectual knowledge and it became increasingly clear that a person's character and social status could no longer claim total precedence over intellectual capabilities. Nevertheless, both forms of militarism survived within the military and civilian sectors of British society. The concept of military efficiency affected all strands of industry, commerce and public service, while the neo-feudalist legacy of 'character over intellect' was largely responsible for the perpetuation of outdated apprenticeship systems. As Cotgrove has argued, 'the traditions of British industry were against the use of academic knowledge and in favour of skill and experience learnt on the job, even on the part of senior management'.[12] In this context, militarism within civilian nursing development reflected far broader trends within British society.

Although military values achieved a high level of popularity within civilian circles, many left-wing MPs expressed considerable doubts regarding these values. The concept of military efficiency and emphasis on the importance of a person's character were not necessarily considered deleterious for society. However, military ideology also incorporated a value system that undermined racial harmony and notions of egalitarianism, since racism was inherent within both aristocratic and technocratic forms of militarism. Similarly, military organisation endorsed social distinctions and a rigid class structure, while the nature of service discipline exuded a form of social control over a person's working and private life.

In view of these military prejudices, the pacifist left within the Attlee Government argued that militarism would eventually corrupt civil society.[13] Discussing the issue of conscription, left-wing representative Tom Scollan remarked that 'it is an evil thing to hand over the youth of the country to the militarist people to be trained in the Army'.[14] There was also the well-founded belief that military conscription would be detrimental to civil society in terms of policy formulation and resource allocation. Nevertheless, others argued that the armed forces supplied an ideal vehicle for social change. It was clearly acknowledged, for instance, that young men would achieve high standards of fitness by conforming to a military lifestyle. Furthermore, many MPs argued that within civil society 'military values such as discipline were intrinsically desirable'.[15] The militarisation of civilian social structures therefore developed by means of a tacit agreement based on an assumption that military values were not only correct but also appropriate for the civilian population. However, while it is possible to acknowledge the existence of militarisation, measuring the intensity of this process is fraught with difficulties. Clearly, an examination of defence expenditure has provided one method of measuring militarisation.

Table 1.1 G-7: defence expenditure as % of GDP, selected years, 1950-80

	1950	1955	1960	1965	1970	1975	1980
Canada	2.6	6.3	4.2	2.9	2.4	1.9	1.8
France	*5.5*	*6.4*	*6.5*	*5.2*	*4.2*	*3.8*	*4.0*
Germany	4.4	4.1	4.0	4.3	3.3	3.6	3.3
Italy	*4.3*	*3.7*	*3.3*	*3.3*	*2.7*	*2.5*	*2.4*
Japan	n.a.	1.8	1.1	0.9	0.8	1.0	1.0
UK	*6.6*	*8.2*	*6.5*	*5.9*	*4.8*	*4.9*	*5.1*
US	5.1	10.2	9.0	7.6	8.0	5.9	5.6
G-7 average	*4.8*	*5.8*	*4.9*	*4.3*	*3.7*	*3.4*	*3.3*

Source: Derived from M. Chalmers, Paying for Defence: Military Spending and British Decline (1985), p.113.

Table 1.1 confirms that the British military received comparatively high amounts of funding in relation to other countries in order to sustain an over-ambitious foreign policy.[16] However, while economic figures have confirmed high levels of British militarism, they do not give any indication of the more insidious forms of militarism.

Since militarisation had wide-ranging effects on all sections of society, an assessment of its impact on social structures entails an examination of civil-military relations. Significantly, accounts of military history have failed to address the ways in which military values were transmitted to civil society. Furthermore, as George and Wilding have observed, 'the study of social policy has contained virtually no analysis of what is meant by social values'.[17] Consequently, the influences affecting social values and structures have rarely been called into question. While militarism provided only one such influence, this study will demonstrate that it was clearly a very important one.

Historical Background

In order to appreciate the significance of military influence on the civilian nursing profession from 1939 onwards, it is necessary to briefly consider the historical background of nursing development prior to this period. For much of the 19th century British nursing lacked a clear professional identity. The sick were cared for more often by relatives and friends than by individuals in possession of recognisable nursing skills. Additional care was provided when necessary by religious sisterhoods and domestic handywomen. Military nursing was predominantly a male domain as women were considered too delicate to care for severely injured men. During the Crimean War the War Office did permit a party of female nurses, led by Florence Nightingale, to nurse the troops in Scutari. The War Office viewed this move as an experiment and, despite the myths that have surrounded the Nightingale legend, it did not fully endorse a commitment to female nursing until after the Boer War. Nightingale had, however, provided the initial breakthrough necessary for the formation and expansion of a female military nursing service. Moreover, the Nightingale Fund[18] established nurse training schools at Netley and at St Thomas's Hospital. Consequently, military and civilian nursing sectors became inextricably linked. However, these training schools did not truly reflect Nightingale's ideas because, while she had appreciated the difficulties associated with nurse training in terms of scope and direction, hospitals adopted only the features inherent in the military system which would result in the formation of a compliant workforce. With what became known as the Nightingale system, the foundations were provided for a coherent secular form of nurse training which had been widely adopted by the turn of the century.

The military values, or militarism, incorporated into the Nightingale system revolved around a sense of duty, self-sacrifice, discipline and respect for authority. As Abel-Smith observed:

> *Over the nurses themselves the matron wielded absolute power. This power was reinforced by the paramilitary organisation of the nursing staff and the rigid discipline imposed in the training schools.* [19]

The bullying tactics frequently employed by matrons and sisters to control probationary nurses also originated within military realms. As the official history of the Royal College of Nursing acknowledged:

> *Naturally only the girls and women who were dedicated to nursing would endure conditions which were exacerbated by a*

tradition of constant bullying and purposeful fault-finding by the sisters. This had its parallel in the ranks of the Regular Army, and it was upon Army traditions and customs that Florence Nightingale had founded skilled nursing. [20]

Since nurses needed to conform to Victorian ideas regarding class and gender, nurses' homes were established to provide a respectable cultural environment for middle-class women although, as Baly has noted, these homes 'all too often became an adjacent barracks, built because it was the cheapest way of housing the labour force that was required to work round the clock for seven days a week'.[21] Moreover, despite the fact that Nightingale had advocated one portal of entry for nurse training, hospitals favoured a two-tiered system. The emerging profession was thus divided between middle- and upper-class lady pupils who paid for their instruction and avoided the more menial nursing duties, and the working-class girls who worked their passage by performing most of the domestic tasks and contributing longer hours of work than their middle-class colleagues. Elitist recruitment practices[22] pursued by the military nursing sector spilled over into the civilian field and, while the military obtained royal patronage for their nursing units, civilian hospitals sought to enhance status by emphasising their own military traditions and reputations. By the turn of the century the nursing profession was clearly dominated by middle-class women, and the social affiliations of the nursing elite mirrored those of the military elite.

However, military influence was not confined to nursing spheres during this period but reflected the wider 'jingoistic' militarism prevalent in British society as a whole. This form of militarism was underpinned by a structural belief system that stressed the importance of the monarchy, religious values, elitism and the aristocratic tradition. In addition, the neo-feudalist military stance, which emphasised the importance of character over intellect, reinforced the relationship between the civilian ruling class and the military elite. As Correlli Barnett has noted, in Great Britain the 'preference for character over intellect took the form of the denigration of the staff college graduate and apotheosis of that splendid chap, the regimental officer'.[23] Since the neo-feudalist stance regarding education was incorporated into nurse training, the belief that 'nurses and midwives were born not made' became perhaps the most stubborn of all stereotypes.[24] Nurses appeared eager to endorse this stereotype and, as a result, nurse training tended to focus exclusively on practical nursing procedures and ignored the potential value of theoretical education. However, while the Nightingale system had constructed a nursing image linked to military authority, this system did not challenge the sexual divisions of labour. Nurses remained subordinate to male physicians. Furthermore, 19th century nursing also incorporated middle-class notions of femininity, religious philanthropy and elements of domestic service. The emergence of militarism as a dominant force was associated primarily with the search for professional status.

Concern with nurse status was motivated not only by the desire to escape the dubious 'Mrs Gamp' image,[25] but also to provide adequate safeguards for patients. The general consensus of nursing opinion recognised the need for professional status but failed to agree on how best to achieve this goal. Was status to be based on social class, religious martyrdom, domestic servitude or military authority? Politically, nurses divided into two camps: those who followed the Nightingale line argued that the status rested on the elite standing of the training hospital, while others, led by a Mrs Bedford Fenwick, pressed for state recognition by means of nurse registration. Nightingale placed great emphasis on the generalist aspect of nursing practice while Bedford Fenwick had advocated the need for specialism.

As nursing evolved, professional organisation emerged. The College of Nursing initially reflected the views of Nightingale supporters, while the Royal British Nurses Association adopted the policies of Bedford Fenwick.[26] However, as College policy eventually shifted direction, both groups pursued the goal of nurse registration. With the exception of asylum workers, all nurses shared similar middle-class backgrounds and professional objectives. The predominantly male working-class content of the asylum labour force placed greater emphasis on promotional structures and wage claims. Despite overtures from asylum workers to join forces with mainstream nursing organisations, the elitist membership of the latter precluded amalgamation and nursing therefore organised in different directions, with inherent divisions of class and gender obscuring the more fundamental issues.

Significantly, the drive towards registration was closely associated with the suffrage movement. War nursing in particular gave added impetus to the claims for citizenship. As Summers has argued, it was thought that 'women's necessary services in war demonstrated their de facto equality with men and their right to franchise'[27] although, ironically, while women viewed military nursing as a vital contribution to the overall war effort, male conscientious objectors within the Royal Army Medical Corps considered war nursing in terms of participating in a life-affirming service. Idealism relating to military involvement soon gave way to realism:

> *Nurses such as Mrs Bedford Fenwick had thought that the*
> *military needs of the state would produce the most convincing*

> *arguments in favour of uniform professional standards in nursing; but in fact the war had shown how easily the state could override the nurses' criteria of professionalism by diluting hospital staffs with barely-trained VADs.* [28]

Nevertheless, the 1918 Representation of the Peoples Act sent another clear message to women; by denying the vote to conscientious objectors the Act underpinned the relationship between war service and legitimate claims for citizenship, although the introduction of female nursing into military realms in the 19th century had been seen as a move towards 'feminising a masculine occupation and civilianising a military institution'.[29] As nurses began to associate citizenship with masculinity and military service, this trend was reversed - nurses became masculinised and civilians militarised.

The thirty-year battle for nurse registration was finally won in 1919, but state recognition did not lead to professionalisation and uniform standards of training failed to emerge. Politically, nurses remained fragmented and failure to agree on policy formulation resulted in government intervention and the creation of the General Nursing Council.[30] Thus:

> *By its own folly the profession had handed over the control of the standard of entry and the requirements for basic training to the government and of course to the ultimate control by people who had the responsibility for keeping the hospitals staffed as cheaply as possible.* [31]

Registration for general nursing entailed a three-year training programme in an approved training school followed by a written and oral examination. In theory, the General Nursing Council was able to withdraw approval from training schools that failed to reach an acceptable standard; in practice, hospitals simply appealed to the Ministry of Health to have the GNC decision overturned. Since the staffing of hospitals was paramount and training only a secondary consideration, the Ministry continually overruled GNC policy on training and educational matters. At all levels of nursing, concern regarding status intensified as the GNC frequently endorsed policies that were economically driven rather than professionally motivated.

Falling recruitment figures and high wastage rates during the inter-war period indicated that young girls no longer viewed nursing as a popular career option, and by 1932:

Over 51% of hospitals were experiencing difficulty in recruiting staff nurses. One third of probationers were not finishing their training and 78% of those were leaving within the first year. [32]

Nursing organisations had failed to assume control of curriculum developments and, while the College emerged as the dominant political force, its professional objectives were severely constrained by material conditions.

Since registered status was not reinforced by professionalism it became increasingly vulnerable to attack. Moreover, the Nightingale system had ossified, leaving little scope for improvements in working conditions or nursing practice. Long hours, poor pay, petty restrictions and compulsory living-in all served as disincentives to recruitment. The nursing elite had believed that to some extent registered status would compensate for poor conditions and the lack of material gain. However, this assumption was not borne out by facts and by 1939 British nursing services were in a state of crisis.

Sources

Much of the primary research material for this study has been obtained from the Public Records Office and, in particular, the files of the Ministry of Health, Ministry of Labour, War Office, the General Nursing Council and the Treasury. However, due to the thirty-year rule of access, some research information was not available, such as material relating to the implementation of Salmon reforms from 1969 onwards. To compensate for this, interviews have been recorded with Brian Salmon CBE and senior nurses involved with the official enquiry. Moreover, some documentation unavailable from the Public Record Office has been obtained from the Royal College of Nursing archives. Contemporary journals and newspapers have also been useful in this respect, as has Hansard.

Research analysis on civilian nursing has been supplemented by records held in hospital archives, particularly medical and nursing minutes and matrons' reports. This material was not widespread; some hospitals failed to keep records of nursing minutes and others only kept them for a limited period of time. The focus of research was therefore dictated by the availability of material. Those hospital records consulted include: Warneford Hospital Archives, Oxford; Bristol Royal Infirmary, Bristol Record Office; Royal London Hospital Archives; Great Ormond Street Hospital Archives; Westminster and St Bartholomews. In addition, some material was obtained for Newcastle and Glasgow. Oral history transcripts pertaining to Manchester Royal Infirmary were also consulted. More general information regarding nurse staffing records was gained from the Modern Records Centre, Warwick. This centre also supplied the official records of the Confederation of Health Service Employees, National Union of Public Employees and the National Association of Local Government Officers.

More detailed research on military nursing has concentrated on archival sources held in the Imperial War Museum and the Queen Alexandra's Royal Army Nursing Corps Museum. However, strict censorship rules governed the nature of military correspondence, so strategic positions and staffing levels were not always revealed. Clearly, some records were destroyed as a direct result of military activity, although individual letters did yield valuable information regarding wartime attitudes and post-war expectations. Since records relating to military nursing gradually decline in number from 1945 onwards, in order to assess the divergence between civilian and military nursing services, interviews were conducted with the Matron-in-Chief of the Armed Forces, Miss Jane Titley (retired 1995) and Colonel E.E. Gruber von Arni RRCL/QARANC, Royal Army Medical College. Additional information was obtained from the Royal United Services and Royal Army Medical Corps Journals.

Structure

This study examines the impact of military influence on civilian nursing development from the outbreak of war in 1939 until the restructuring of nurse administration in 1969. The book attempts to explain how and why military influence proved to be instrumental in preventing nurse reform. Initially, however, it is necessary to explore the role of nurses within the 'warfare-welfare' state. The second chapter, therefore, will assess the relationship between military and civilian nurses and discuss the overall impact of war on the British nursing services, while subsequent chapters will focus on nursing development from 1945 onwards.

Since the text follows a thematic rather than a strict chronological structure, research material is frequently chronologically uneven within these chapters, though analysis will explore the myriad of ways in which militarism infiltrated basic nursing care and prevented reform. It is hoped that, to some extent at least, this military influence can be measured and evaluated since, although aspects of militarism can be detected within the histories of many civilian professions and organisations, British nursing history provides the clearest example of how militarism in its various forms has consistently impinged on civilian social structures.

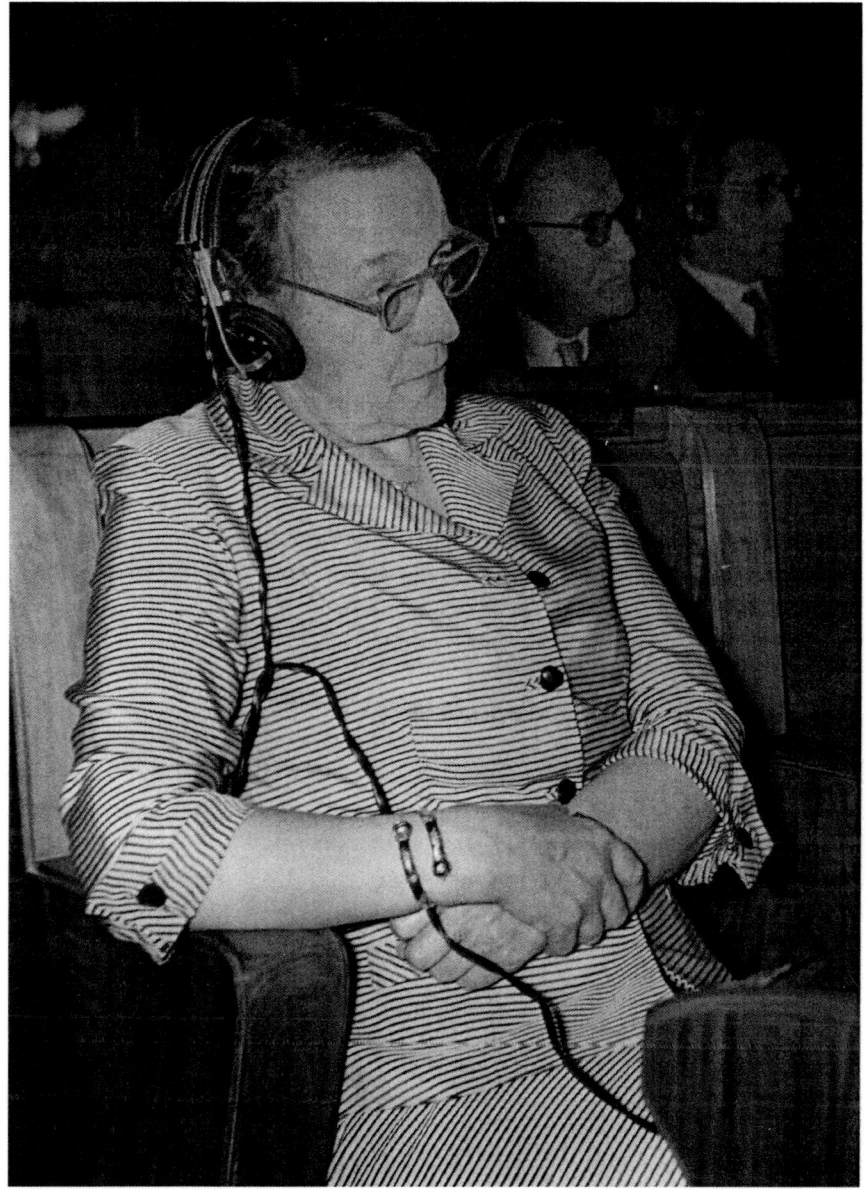

Dame Elizabeth Cockayne, Minister of Health, one of the main speakers at the technical discussions on nurses, their education and their role in health programmes at the Ninth World Health Assembly, Geneva 1956.

End Notes

(1)   A. Summers, *Angels and Citizens* (1988), p.295
(2)   M. Shaw, *Post Military Society* (1991), p.118
(3)   V.R. Berghann, *Militarism: the history of an international debate* (Cambridge, 1981), p.108
(4)   *Ibid.*, p.105
(5)   *Ibid.*, p.106
(6)   Berghann, *op cit.*, p.116
(7)   Shaw, *op cit.*, p.12
(8)   C. Enloe, *The Morning After: sexual politics in the Cold War* (1993)
(9)   Shaw, *op cit.*, p.113
(10)   *Ibid.*, p.118
(11)   *Ibid.*, p.113
(12)   S. Cotgrove, *Technical Education and Social Change: first Annual Report of the Advisory Council on Scientific Policy*, Cmd 7465 (1948), p.15
(13)   L.V. Scott, *Conscription and the Attlee Government* (1993), p.139
(14)   *Ibid.*
(15)   *Ibid.*, p.95
(16)   Clearly, military personnel were also dictating policy formulation. A threatened resignation by Military Chiefs of Staff for example was instrumental in maintaining a British role in the Middle East.
(17)   V. George and P. Wilding, *Social Values and Social Class* (1972), p.236
(18)   The Nightingale Fund was set up as a charity by a 'grateful public'. The money was used to establish a civilian nurse training school at St Thomas's Hospital in London and a military nurse training school at Netley. Neither of the training schools fully incorporated Nightingale's ideas.
(19)   B. Abel-Smith, *A History of the Nursing Profession* (1960), p.29
(20)   C. Bowman, *The Lamp and the Book* (1966), p.105
(21)   M. Baly, *Nursing and Social Change* (1980), p.133
(22)   The military nursing services recruited primarily from the ranks of officers' wives or widows, and ladies from the higher echelons of society.
(23)   C. Barnett, 'The Education of the Military Elite', in R. Wilkinson, ed., *Governing Elites* (Oxford, 1969), p.196
(24)   A. Briggs, *The Briggs Committee Report on the Nursing Services* (1972), p.31
(25)   Mrs Gamp was a character created by Charles Dickens who portrayed nurses as gin-soaked women with little if any nursing skill.
(26)   There were numerous nursing organisations, but the College of Nursing became the largest and most influential. It was founded in 1916 by Sir Arthur Stanley.
(27)   Summers, *op cit.*, p.182
(28)   *Ibid.*, p.90
(29)   *Ibid.*, p.28
(30)   For background of General Nursing Council, see Abel-Smith, *op cit.*
(31)   Baly, *op cit.*, p.162
(32)   C. Hart, *Behind the Mask* (1994), p.55

Chapter 2

Fighting Militarism?
British Nursing during the Second World War

On a fundamental level, nursing aims from 1939 onwards were twofold: firstly, to administer adequate nursing care to their patients; and secondly, to protect and enhance professional status. These aims were not compatible. Wartime chaos was compounded by inept government policy and the nursing services were diluted with untrained personnel the instant war broke out. Within a matter of weeks the healthcare needs of civilians were subordinated to those of the emergency services.[1] Staff at voluntary hospitals were conscripted and subjected to the jurisdiction of the Ministry of Health, and the outpatient departments of such hospitals disappeared virtually overnight. Figures estimated that 10 million patients attended these hospitals every year, and the absence of outpatient clinics placed a substantial burden on the district nursing services. The government introduced an Emergency Hospital Scheme that divided the country into sectors, with a matron and administrative staff responsible for each sector, and established first aid posts to assist with casualty clearance.[2] But the need to recruit, train and deploy nurses in adequate numbers for the duration of war presented the government with a problem that was never fully resolved.

Disincentives to nurse recruitment had been identified by a government committee chaired by the Earl of Athlone, and the Athlone Interim Report published in 1939[3] suggested that a two-pronged approach would improve the situation. Firstly, it was suggested that the government should afford official recognition to assistant nurses, and secondly, that voluntary hospitals should be subsidised to enable them to standardise training and improve salaries These modest recommendations were initially rejected by both government and nursing camps. Registered nurses objected to the proposed recognition of assistant nurses as they believed this would downgrade their professional status, while government officials opposed the idea of funding voluntary hospitals. Yet as the war progressed, both government and nursing camps were forced to make concessions. These same concessions provided the somewhat dubious foundations for post-war nursing organisation.

Throughout the war, government and, in some instances, hospital officials demonstrated a remarkable level of ignorance regarding nursing issues. Recruitment was viewed merely in terms of overall figures with no regard for the proficiency levels of individual nursing grades, and government policy towards healthcare delivery was frequently ill-conceived. As the nursing profession attempted to establish a sense of order from wartime chaos and expand its sphere of influence in the process,[4] it was concern over nurse status that dominated professional thinking. Military nurses strove to resolve the ambiguity of their position within the armed forces, while civilian nurses tried desperately to enhance their professional status and abandon the image of motherhood. Both groups adopted militarisation strategies in order to achieve these goals, but with varying degrees of success. These strategies incorporated military customs and ideals into everyday nursing practice and, in order to establish the origins and popularity of such overt military identification, this militarisation process will be discussed at length. Furthermore, it will be argued that militarisation exerted a detrimental effect on patient care, hindered the professionalisation of nursing and contained significant implications for the reconstruction of post-war nursing services. In the first instance, however, since militarisation was prompted by the erosion of registered nurse status, it is important to examine the ways in which this status was undermined.

Status Undermined

Registered nurse status was undermined in three key areas from 1939 onwards: firstly, in the way in which nursing services were organised; secondly, by recruitment and training procedures; and thirdly, by government legislation. It is necessary, therefore, to examine these three areas in some depth.

Organisation

Initial attempts to organise the medical services in preparation for war were ill-conceived, inefficient and heavily criticised by members of the medical profession. In the government White Paper of July 1939, the Ministry of Health had outlined a system of first aid posts, with the intention that all such posts would be staffed by a qualified doctor with trained nurses in attendance. Many of London's voluntary hospitals were to act as casualty clearing stations and plans were unveiled to disperse a proportion of the population living in major cities to surrounding rural areas. There were, however, fundamental problems associated with these emergency plans. To begin with, there were not enough trained doctors and nurses to staff the first aid posts. Then there was the problem of medical 'specialism'. Doctors who were available to staff such first aid posts were not necessarily experienced in orthopaedic surgery and many did not possess the medical skills required to deal with air raid casualties. There was also some dispute between medical personnel and government officials regarding the method of casualty clearance. To an extent, British emergency schemes for casualty clearance were based on medical experience gained during the Spanish Civil War. The Spanish conflict had provided Britain with a perfect case study, both in terms of observing the effects of modern warfare and the treatment of civilian casualties. Nevertheless, British officials chose to ignore some of the more important medical lessons gained as a result of the Spanish conflict. Professor Trueta, chief of a large surgical unit in Barcelona, had visited England in October 1939 to address the Royal Society of Medicine. The main purpose of his visit was to advise the British medical profession on the treatment of air raid casualties.

Trueta claimed that Spanish experience had shown that unless injuries received immediate 'on the spot' skilled attention, subsequent treatment was very often useless - a medical point which was not fully appreciated by the British Ministry of Health. Skilled surgical teams, Trueta argued, needed to be situated in the centre of all major cities. In view of this advice, Sir Ernest Graham-Little of the University of London had approached the Minister of Health and requested that he 'revise the arrangements by which nearly all the experienced surgeons were waiting for casualties in centres remote from London'.[5] This appeal, however, was ignored. Some officials expressed sympathy with Graham-Little's point of view; there were others though who argued that casualties should be given basic first aid as a temporary measure and transported out of city centres as quickly as possible. There were also those who severely doubted the role of voluntary hospitals within the planned emergency schemes, particularly in London.

As Sir Ralph Wedgwood, Chairman of the Formation Committee of the Air Raid Defence League, argued:

> From almost every aspect, London hospitals are unsuitable for casualty clearing stations. To make them bombproof would be expensive and in most cases impossible. Far too many of our hospitals are liable to attack during an air raid. St Thomas's and Westminster are close to Battersea power station, which will be a target. Others are fatally close to the Thames. [6]

What was needed, Sir Ralph argued, was a network of casualty clearing stations outside London, whereas under the government's emergency scheme casualties were exposed to further danger rather than being transported to an area of safety. This debate on the merits and drawbacks of casualty clearance procedures was largely superfluous since a severe shortage of medical personnel prevented the efficient implementation of any emergency scheme. The shortage of doctors forced medical schools to open their doors to women, and dentists were encouraged to acquire anaesthetic skills by means of intensive courses. A Civil Nursing Reserve (CNR) was established to supplement civilian nursing services, which were considerably depleted since many nurses had volunteered to join the military and territorial services. In addition, the British Red Cross Society and the Order of St John of Jerusalem provided Voluntary Aid Detachment nurses (VADs) to supplement both military and civilian nursing services.[7]

From the outset, however, there were severe difficulties associated with the CNR, many of which originated with the Ministry of Health. For example, the terms and conditions of CNR service were not even published until August 1939 and nurses were understandably reluctant to commit their services to an unknown quantity. Moreover, while the government had formed a Central Emergency Committee for the nursing profession, a body designed to advise the Minister of Health regarding nursing issues and assist with the organisation of reserve nurses, the Committee contained only five trained nurses. Three of these nurses were the Matrons in Chief of the armed forces, preoccupied for the most part with organising their own services rather than the CNR. The remaining nurse members consisted of the Chairman of the GNC and a member of the College of Nursing. By the end of 1939 the Central Emergency Committee was deemed to be a failure. Government officials accused committee members of inefficiency regarding nurse recruitment and allocation, while the national press revealed widespread discontent amongst the nursing population regarding the overall organisation of the CNR. In an attempt to resolve this discontent, the Minister of Health established a Central Advisory Board for Nursing.

The Advisory Board contained fourteen nurse members, mainly representatives of the College, the GNC, the Central Midwives Board, National Council of Nurses, Queen's Institute of District Nurses and the Association of Hospital Matrons.[8] The Board convened on a monthly basis from 1940 onwards and policies were implemented to make the CNR more effective. Nursing officials were appointed for each of the hospital regions to co-ordinate the allocation of reserve nurses. In addition, communications between local medical services and the Ministry of Health were improved. Nevertheless, despite the introduction of these measures, the problems confronting the CNR were far from over.

Initially, reserve nurses assigned to the emergency services were precluded from assisting in other nursing areas, many therefore complained of boredom during the phony war period and abandoned the reserve to seek other employment.[9] Meanwhile, nurses working in tuberculosis hospitals were severely overworked because of staff shortages. The midwifery sector were also experiencing staffing problems along with hospitals for the mentally ill and mentally handicapped. The fact that these hospitals were unable to draw on the resources of the reserve at this stage exposed a major planning weakness. There were also problems associated with levels of nursing expertise. The CNR consisted mainly of assistant nurses and auxiliaries rather than registered nurses. Consequently, registered nurses who had left hospital work to join the armed forces were usually replaced by assistants although, in some cases, this dilution of nursing personnel constituted a deliberate attempt on the part of hospitals to reduce their wage bills. For example, it was estimated that by November 1939 over 2,000 registered nurses had been forced out of their jobs in London and a similar pattern emerged across the country. Hospital administrators had not valued registered nurse status and viewed emergency conditions as an opportunity to save money. In this respect, the way in which reserve nurses were deployed clearly undermined registered status.

The salary discrepancies that existed between regular and reserve nurses also caused severe disruption. Registered nurses working for the CNR were paid the sum of £90 per annum while registered hospital nurses were, on average, paid £70 per annum. Not surprisingly, many hospital nurses left their normal employment to join the reserve. Belated government intervention in 1941 only narrowly averted a complete breakdown in civilian nursing services. During this year the role of the reserve was extended to include all hospitals experiencing severe nursing shortages, and the Ministry of Health stated that regular nurses should be paid the same salary as reserve nurses.[10] Hospitals were not, however, about to implement such a policy without some form of compensation and the Ministry was forced to fund a percentage of the pay difference. The government was now in a position far removed from its pre-war stance. By partially funding nurses in a variety of hospitals the Ministry of Health had become the largest employer of nurses. The CNR, therefore, had provided the foundations for the post-war employer/employee relationship between the Ministry of Health and the nursing profession.

The rift between regular and reserve personnel remained a wartime problem for civilian nursing services, and a similar rift had occurred within the armed forces. The military divide emerged between regular military nurses and those of the Voluntary Aid Detachment. This divide was also fuelled by organisational difficulties. The VAD Council had received numerous complaints from VAD nurses during the early stages of the war, mainly regarding accommodation standards and conditions of service. Several VADs refused to perform some of the more menial nursing tasks and many more objected to sleeping in substandard living quarters. In an attempt to pacify the

VAD Council, the Army Council limited the scope of VAD duties and afforded them officer privileges, concessions which only served to increase the number of arguments relating to nurse status and create anomalies in terms of VAD task allocation.

Qualified nurses resented officer privileges being awarded to VAD nursing assistants. Qualified non-nursing VADs such as opticians and radiographers were disappointed because they were denied these privileges, and male nursing orderlies expressed dissatisfaction at having to perform all the unskilled nursing tasks. The level of discontent amongst military nursing grades escalated since, although VAD nurses enjoyed officer privileges, they were clearly unable to assume officer workloads, neither could these same VADs adequately replace male orderlies. Consequently, when male orderlies were transferred to front line positions as the course of the war altered, VAD task allocation presented considerable strategic problems. The Army Council response to these problems was unprecedented. In 1943, comprehensive proposals were submitted to the War Office aimed at incorporating VADs into the Auxiliary Territorial Service (ATS). The Army claimed that the existing organisational structure was inefficient and did not fully utilise man and woman power. There was considerable justification for this claim. Army officials argued that a number of VADs were capable of undergoing training courses which would equip them for a nursing career in civil society once hostilities ceased. Under the existing scheme VADs were unable to take advantage of certain training opportunities, regardless of their individual abilities. The army proposals were designed to rectify this state of affairs.

It was suggested that the new VAD branch of the ATS would be organised through the ATS record office, as the new branch 'would form an integral part of the ATS and not of the Royal Army Medical Corps or the Army Dental Corps'.[11] This statement reflected Army Council policy regarding female personnel, namely that there should only be one female corps within the army. The army proposals, however, were not merely designed to encourage VAD training and resolve status issues; the proposals made provision for the army to dispense with the services of the VAD Council. Army funds would therefore no longer be awarded to the VAD Council or to VAD county controllers. Furthermore, the army would acquire a substantial nursing force to direct at will.

There were, nevertheless, important flaws inherent within these army takeover plans. Army officials had not, for example, considered the wider implications of a merger between VAD and ATS personnel. Aside from the potential ethical questions associated with a military takeover of voluntary services, the proposals, if accepted, clearly compromised the British Red Cross position within the international arena. If the military could take over Red Cross VADs, then why not their communications and administration? Red Cross principles were based overwhelmingly on the concept of political neutrality. How could this political neutrality co-exist with military compliance regarding voluntary nurses? There was also the potential problem of a loss of 'goodwill'. Voluntary bodies had made concerted efforts to train enough first aiders and nursing aids for wartime service. Given the overall shortage of medical personnel, it was not possible to administer adequate care to civilian and military casualties without continued voluntary assistance. A forced takeover bid of voluntary nurses was not likely to foster good relationships between the state and the voluntary bodies concerned. As Cambray and Briggs have noted, the suggested destruction of 'the oldest women's service met with the most violent resistance from the VADs and societies concerned'.[12] After much deliberation, in June 1943 an ad hoc committee rejected the proposed merger and suggested that, since the treatment of VADs in the armed forces had undermined registered nurse status, 'steps should be taken to avoid the use by VAD members of any articles of clothing which are generally identified with particular ranks of the nursing profession'.[13]

Despite this recommendation, most nurses continued to be preoccupied with their status. Senior nurses argued that status issues were inextricably linked to recruitment issues, thus, if nurse status could not be elevated and maintained, it would not be possible to attract new recruits into the profession. However, in terms of recruitment, another important dimension needed to be added to the nursing equation - that of nurse training.

Training and recruitment

Nurse training techniques had changed little since the days of Nightingale and the introduction of nurse registration in 1919 had failed to produce uniform standards in the education and training of nurses. Registration for general nursing entailed a three-year apprenticeship programme in an approved nurse training school, followed by a written and oral examination. In theory the GNC was able to withdraw approval from training schools which failed to reach an acceptable standard, but hospitals which failed to meet such standards usually appealed to the Ministry of Health to overturn GNC decisions. These appeals were frequently successful since the staffing of hospitals took precedence over training considerations.

In comparison to the civilian sector, nursing orderlies in the Royal Army Medical Corps were subjected to a far more unified and comprehensive training scheme, primarily because the ability to wage war successfully was considered to be a political priority, although both military and civilian training schemes maximised apprentice labour without providing adequate theoretical knowledge. As a former RAMC Class III orderly recalled, experience on the wards was limited to such things as:

> ... bumping the ward floor until it shone like a mirror, cleaning the kitchen, blackleading the fireplace in sister's office, to giving and taking away bedpans and urinals and to cleaning the sluice. Any dressings, medicines etc. were given by the sister or VAD but when showing an interest I was allowed to look.[14]

Nurse training was dictated by hospital demands in the civilian sector and strategic demands in the military sector. Both forms of nurse apprenticeship exuded an anti-educational bias whereby the character-moulding process took precedence over the stimulation of intellect, and there appeared to be a basic assumption within government circles that nursing skills could be equated with mothering skills. The Ministry of Health, along with the Ministry of Labour, for instance, believed that nurses should supervise children in day nurseries to enable more women to work in industry, although:

> Many questioned whether SRNs were the most appropriate people to supervise the under-fives. The matron of a Coventry nursery admitted anxiously that she had plenty of experience but none with healthy children and there were suspicions that nurses tended to leave children in high chairs and play pens with nothing to do. [15]

Registered nurses were eager to abandon this image of motherhood and be recognised as professionals with valuable skills. This ambition was not reflected in the nurse training process since domestic and practical tasks continued to dominate a probationer's training. Registered status also appeared to be a dubious goal as, on completion of training, very little distinction was made between registered and assistant nursing grades in terms of task allocation.

This ongoing lack of distinction between registered and assistant nurses created further status problems. Registered nurses described assistants as 'bath attendants' and asserted their status by recalling tales of heroic military experience, while assistant nurses accused their registered counterparts of snobbery. As one assistant complained in the nursing press:

> *I have no certificate to show for my hard work, but I'll wager if I were to collect my testimonials they would carry me further than some of those people who are so fond of boasting of their registered status and medals.* [16]

Registered nurses, however, viewed their status in terms of the thirty-year struggle for professional recognition, a struggle that had achieved little in the way of uniform standards of training but nonetheless provided a foundation for further professionalisation. The interchangeable nature of the assistant nurse role, along with the demands of war, represented an obvious threat to this professionalisation. A prime example of this threat could be detected within the industrial nursing sector.

The wartime demand for industrial nurses had prompted a substantial reduction in the training period for this qualification, initially reduced from a period of one year to that of nine months, eventually declining to a period of only three months. Eventually, it was also possible to obtain an industrial nurse certificate by undertaking a correspondence course! All of these courses were administered by the College of Nursing and known to be inadequate. This problem was overlooked by government officials, simply because the demand for industrial nurses to work in munitions factories far exceeded supply, despite the fact that the recruitment of nurses for the industrial sector remained vibrant when compared to other civilian nursing fields. Many nurses favoured working in the industrial environment because the hours of work in hospitals were far longer than those worked in the factories. Others gravitated towards industrial work because they were not required to 'live in'. There was, however, a gender divide in terms of recruitment to industrial nursing, with far more men applying to enter this sector than women. Recruitment propaganda specifically targeted men to work as factory nurses since the need to mobilise women for the war effort was balanced continually against the need to maintain a patriarchal society. Industry needed, therefore, to be primarily associated with masculinity rather than femininity, regardless of war.

A further blow to nursing's professional goals came in the form of 'child exploitation'. Inspired by military recruitment practice, 'cadet schemes' were introduced to alleviate nursing shortages. Fifteen-year old girls were recruited directly from school and expected to perform skilled nursing tasks, often without supervision. In some instances cadets were responsible for suturing wounds, attending post mortems and feeding premature babies. These girls were also denied any form of organised training. Civilian cadet schemes were therefore an obvious distortion of the military model of practice. As Encel noted:

> *The professional military model embraces features such as early recruitment, the specialised training of cadets in a separate college, careful career planning, and post-graduate work in a staff college.*[17]

Clearly, the civilian model had failed to incorporate these features. Cadets in some areas attended college one day a week, but they were taught subjects which were unrelated to their work environment.[18]

Despite their lack of training, cadets became adept at performing skilled nursing tasks, which presented a significant problem for registered nurses. How could a three-year training period be justified for registration, if fifteen-year-old girls were able to acquire nursing skills with no training whatsoever? Improved recruitment levels in the form of cadet schemes, therefore, ultimately undermined the position of the registered nurse. This process was also assisted by government legislation.

Government policy

With regard to the nursing profession, policies that emanated from the Ministry of Health from 1939 onwards established a pattern which continued for decades. This pattern emphasised that overall concern was for quantity of nurses rather than quality. In an attempt to obtain this quantity, the government abolished the minimum educational qualification for nurse training in 1939. Recruitment procedures paid little attention to the level of experience of nurses accepted for military service and, until 1943, the intake of nurses into the armed forces was unrestricted. When combined with the disjointed Civil Nursing Reserve, this unrestricted flow of nurses into the forces created severe chaos. Most civilian hospitals were unable to replace the senior nurses who had volunteered for military service and consequently, in 1941, steps were taken by the War Office to return senior nurses to their respective hospitals on request, if the institutions concerned were experiencing difficulties in filling senior positions. These steps were ineffective. The time lapse between making a request to the War Office and receiving the released nurse tended to be a period of at least six months. Military nurses were often overseas and therefore difficult to locate and recall at short notice.

Civilian health services were badly disrupted by this shortage of senior nurses, particularly in areas such as midwifery, tuberculosis and mental nursing. The government had afforded priority to military healthcare services in order to achieve military objectives but, as the voluntary services pointed out, 'civil defence workers were in the most literal sense in the front line'.[19] Nevertheless, government officials failed to provide any healthcare facilities for these workers. It was left to the war organisation of the Red Cross and St John to step into the brink and establish a 'Rest House' scheme for civil defence workers, although their efforts were not fully appreciated by members of the public. 'An impression arose that it was a way of providing 'free holidays' for a class of hale and hearty civilians who were subjected to no greater strain than others in civil life' - a view disputed by Lord Horder, who described the scheme as a 'piece of pioneering work in preventative medicine'.[20]

The government failed to match this voluntary initiative and local authorities were not permitted under the Civil Defence Acts of 1937 and 1939 to incur expenditure in supplying welfare facilities for civil defence personnel. Although members of the voluntary services were 'somewhat surprised that government took so negative a view of its welfare responsibilities',[21] nurses were not surprised. They believed that government officials were oblivious to welfare issues and, for many, this view was confirmed by the controversial Nurses Act of 1943. In essence, the legislation only served to legitimise existing practice by giving official recognition to assistant nurses, and was primarily designed to aid recruitment. But the Act was also prompted by a need to reassure the public that they were being nursed by qualified personnel.

Government officials believed that since a shortage of registered nurses had resulted in the widespread employment of assistants, some legislation was necessary to convince the public that these assistants were trained nurses. This action in itself was enough to provoke hostility from registered nurses. However, the Act also stated that the administration of assistants should be funded by nurse registration fees. To add insult to injury, a clause was included in the Act that allowed Christian Science nurses to assume the official title of 'nurse' without possessing any relevant skills. The profession was appalled. As the nursing press proclaimed:

> *It is almost incredible that after the profession of nursing has existed in England for a quarter of a century, that totally ignorant Ministers of the Crown should be permitted to smash up not only the status of an honourable profession but deprive the public of necessary safeguards to health and life.* [22]

Senior nurses at the GNC and College of Nursing adopted a pragmatic approach and sanctioned the Act, but for many registered nurses the legislation represented an outright betrayal of their professional ideals.

Status Regained?

As the erosion of registered nurse status continued unabated, some members of the profession attempted to retrieve the situation. The virtual collapse of nursing services during the early stages of war had prompted government officials to seek nursing advice, and in 1941 senior nursing appointments were established at the Ministry of Health, Ministry of Labour and the Colonial Office in an effort to create a more substantial and cohesive nursing service. Senior nurses installed in Whitehall were expected to resolve some of the long-standing problems associated with nurse recruitment. Despite government expectations, however, 'the number of permanent trained staff remained static throughout the war at 23,000-24,000'[23] and, in view of the stability of these figures, it would be tempting to assume that additional trained nurses simply did not exist. In fact, there were over 80,000 nurses registered with the GNC in 1939. It is not clear from official records whether the 9,000 registered nurses serving with the armed forces were included in the original figure of 24,000. If they were excluded, then the original estimate would reach that of 33,000. Therefore, if these figures are to be believed, at least 47,000 trained nurses had opted out of the profession. It should be noted that the GNC register was not always kept up to date in terms of available nurses[24] but, nonetheless, the main aim in terms of nurse recruitment centred on the need to persuade trained nurses to return to their profession.

In 1943, with this aim in mind, a government appointed committee chaired by Lord Rushcliffe attempted to woo trained nurses. In essence, Rushcliffe merely resurrected the earlier findings of the 1939 Athlone Interim Report. National pay scales that reflected the divergence between trained and untrained staff were hastily introduced, along with the recommendation of a 96-hour fortnight for all nurses. Moreover, in order to improve the distribution of nurses, the Control of Engagement Order, which had applied to women aged between 18 and 40 years of age since 1942, was extended to include nurses in 1943. In addition, the government implemented measures to restrict the intake of nurses into the armed forces. Certain categories of nurses, previously considered eligible for military service, were now exempt. These included hospital matrons, assistant matrons and sister tutors, practising midwives and health visitors, practising district nurses and nurses employed in sanatoria, experienced sick children's nurses and mental nurses. In cases of severe nursing shortages, hospitals were also permitted to request the postponement of 'call-up' with regard to nurses not included in the aforementioned categories.[25]

The combination of these measures provided a 'carrot and stick' approach to nursing problems. Senior nurses were convinced that the improved salary scales implemented as a result of Rushcliffe would improve professional status, particularly since these scales emphasised the difference between trained and untrained staff. However, as Baly has noted, 'this sudden economic improvement, some nurses doubling their salaries, made almost no difference to the recruitment figures',[26] although the improved salaries may have prevented a more serious exodus of existing nurses. Regardless of his intentions to improve nurse recruitment in the sanatoria and mental nursing fields, Rushcliffe actually contributed to severe nursing shortages since the introduction of national pay scales prevented hospitals from offering pay incentives, which were necessary to attract nurses to work in isolated areas. There were further reasons for the ultimate failure of Rushcliffe to ease the nursing situation.

By the time Rushcliffe pay scales were introduced, the cost of living had risen by over 40%, which largely negated the effects of salary improvements. Nurses were also dismayed by a GNC decision to extend the period of registered training to that of four years instead of three. The GNC maintained that a longer training period would have the effect of enhancing nurse status, thus improving nurse recruitment. However, since Rushcliffe had widened the pay differentials between trained and untrained staff, the GNC decision was clearly dictated by economic considerations. The 1943 Nurses Act had tightened government control over nursing issues and, as the largest employer of nurses, the Ministry of Health had a vested interest in promoting policies which were economically driven rather than professionally motivated. The GNC had become the mouthpiece of the Ministry, and State intervention in professional matters had served to alienate nurses, although a training exemption within the Control of Engagement Order was exploited to the full. Over 90% of newly qualified nurses chose to embark on further training courses rather than to have their work dictated by the Minister of Labour. This trend effectively limited the impact of nursing controls but at least alleviated shortages in the midwifery sector by encouraging more nurses to undertake midwifery training. Nursing shortages generally, and in particular the lack of trained staff, continued to cause problems for healthcare delivery. Because nurses opted for further training on qualifying, the overall ratio of trained to untrained staff was adversely affected. Indeed, despite Rushcliffe's efforts to improve status by salary increases, it was still possible for women to earn more money for fewer hours in munitions factories.

Restricting the intake of nurses into the armed forces had also compounded problems from a military viewpoint. As Britain began waging war on a 'second front' in 1944, the demand for nurses increased dramatically. The restrictions on nurse conscription were therefore extremely ill-timed. On occasions the shortage of military nurses led to 'a force of 2,000 QAs nursing under stress extra beds to the tune of twelve thousand'.[27] These nursing shortages were particularly severe in the Far East. More importantly, the services were now encumbered with very inexperienced nurses rather than the highly trained nurses of previous years.

The organisation of military medical services had already been hampered by problems associated with VAD task allocation, although it is not clear from official records whether the ad hoc committee set up to resolve VAD problems was timed to coincide with government restrictions on nurse intake. The VAD Council was substituted with a standing committee that incorporated the Council of Territorial Associations along with representatives from the various voluntary organisations. The ad hoc committee, as previously acknowledged, had gone some way to resolving nurse status issues, but the nursing position vis-a-vis the women's services was far from clear. The army had decided to incorporate only one women's service. If the Auxiliary Territorial Service (ATS) were established as a corps, where did this leave military nurses? How would the military nursing position be defined in the post-war years? How would nursing as a whole compete with other forms of employment if professional status could not be enhanced and protected? Clearly, the profession desperately needed to raise nurse status and, since the demands of war precluded the enhancement of prestige by professional means, nurses sought an alternative route.

Militarisation

For a profession with strong military roots, it was not uncharacteristic for civilian nurses to be identified with the armed forces. It was also not uncommon for military nurses to be obsessed with rank and the trappings of military customs prior to the Second World War. One pre-war naval nurse recalled that 'The mess was very rank conscious - the laundry matron used to hang out our dresses in order of rank'.[28] Civilian nursing too had adopted many of the petty restrictions associated with military protocol. As a consequence of these civil-military connections, recruitment propaganda from 1939 onwards concentrated on nursing's heroic and military past. A film that charted the life of First World War heroine Edith Cavell raised £62,000 for the British Red Cross Society and gave impetus to the recruitment drive in the early stages of war.[29] A similar film, entitled *The Lamp Still Burns*, highlighted the self-effacing heroism of nurses.[30] The Ministry of Health capitalised on this heroic trend in recruitment posters. As one poster asserted:

> *In every war in our history, Britain has looked to the women to care for the sick and wounded. It is women's work. The nurses never let us down. Florence Nightingale lit a candle in the Crimea 85 years ago. The women of today have kept it burning brightly not only in France, Egypt and Greece but in Poplar, Portsmouth, Liverpool, Hull and all other battlefields of the Home Front.* [31]

These military and heroic overtones with regard to nurses, however, formed part of a wider militarisation process within society, a time when even librarians donned military style uniforms. This overall trend served to blur the dividing line between militarisation as a 'natural' process of war and militarisation as a deliberate policy with specific aims and objectives.

The proliferation of civilian nurse cadet schemes, for instance, could be attributed to a more general tendency towards military identification. It can also be argued that frequent requests to the Ministry of Health by midwives eager to wear military uniforms also reflected the wider militarisation process. However, in addition to the overall trend, militarisation did emerge as a distinct and deliberate nursing policy. The leading protagonist of this policy was Dame Katherine Jones[32] who, as Matron in Chief of the army, argued that militarisation provided an opportunity to resolve nurse status problems once and for all. The aims of the policy were threefold: first, to define the nursing position within the armed forces vis-a-vis the women's service; second, to provide a framework that would secure nurse status for the profession as a whole; and finally, to shift the nursing image away from motherhood towards that of masculine military efficiency.

Nurses within the army were already afforded nominal officer status and, since the Nightingale era, were recruited primarily from the ranks of officers' wives, widows and daughters. Elitist recruitment practice combined with royal patronage ensured that military nursing occupied a prestigious position within the profession as a whole. Despite this prestige, however, the nursing position within the army was always ambiguous. This position was described by Summers as being 'in but not of the Army'.[33] Female military nursing units had existed since the Crimea and were not disbanded along with other female military units in 1918.[34] Nevertheless, with the onset of the Second World War, when compared with other female units, the nursing position had declined both in terms of status and pay.

Members of the ATS had adopted a policy of military assimilation in order to secure their status and Dame Katherine believed that nurses could also benefit from such a policy. The ATS had recognised that militarisation provided the key which enabled women to gain commissioned officer status. As Dame Katherine observed:

> *The ATS officer achieved that understanding from the start. It was reinforced by a multitude of detailed practices, it was emphasised by the cut and the colour of her uniform and there was no doubt at any point that she fitted into the army pattern. She was recognised everywhere by everyone as an army officer both on and off duty. It became my aim to profit from this experience and to achieve the same assimilation for the QAIMNS.* [35]

More importantly, Dame Katherine argued that if registered nurses in the military sector obtained commissioned officer status, this would to some extent elevate and promote nurse status in the civilian sector. As she explained to the Association of Hospital Matrons (AHM):

> *I want you to understand this as the imposition of the military rank pattern on the nursing profession. By superimposing this rank pattern on one particular section of the nursing profession, it seemed possible to not only confer status but to provide a framework to hold that status firmly in place.* [36]

With this goal in mind, the Matron in Chief initiated a full-blown militarisation programme for army nurses.

The process of military assimilation involved identification with masculinity and a corresponding suppression of the more feminine aspects of nursing. Nurses were expected to stress the concept of efficiency as this was considered to be a military virtue. Fitness programmes were introduced and nurses were increasingly expected to administer care in front line positions. One nurse described this transition:

> *Until this stage we sisters had never been drilled, suddenly we found ourselves forming fours and route marching three miles into the desert and back, all to get us fit for the Greek episode.* [37]

Another nurse, writing in 1942, described her feelings with regard to the front line policy:

Waiting for the baptism of fire doesn't worry me much except for the usual empty feeling at the sound of planes and guns. One sister here has been through France, the Middle East and Greece with amazing experiences and I want to do likewise. At last my existence here seems justified and the year of fun and games preceding this will be something to be remembered with a tolerant smile. [38]

Some nurses clearly did view the introduction of route marches and drill procedures as 'fun and games'. Others, however, took the militarisation process very seriously. In some cases patients were allocated beds and examined by medical officers according to their rank. The lowest rank was always the last to receive medical attention, irrespective of the severity of illness and injury. Not everyone shared this overt enthusiasm for militarisation. For instance, Commonwealth nurses, particularly Australians, claimed that British nurses were obsessed with status, rank and protocol.

Despite the resistance of Commonwealth nurses, militarisation continued. Army nurses' uniforms were changed from the traditional scarlet and grey to that of khaki and, for the first time, their uniform included a 'battle dress'. These changes represented the tangible effects of militarisation. The more insidious effects, such as the adoption of military values with regard to social class and race, were less immediately apparent. These values were the supposed virtues and superiority of the British Empire and the importance of social and racial hierarchy. Undoubtedly, nursing attitudes were influenced by the inculcation of these values, as their correspondence reveals. One nurse stated of her experience in Benghazi:

Our batmen were an education to us in themselves. The majority of them had obviously been swinging from tree to tree in the jungles of India until only a few weeks previously. [39]

Another, writing from Baghdad, declared that:

Everyone has heard of the thief of Baghdad. We discovered that he has thousands of descendants. The Baghdad Iraqi, like most town Arabs, is out to 'do' his own grandmother and, since we couldn't claim even this relationship, we didn't stand a chance! A trial 'black out' took place soon after our arrival but it proved such a godsend to the local gentry, who took the opportunity to murder and steal with great gusto, that it was thought that even a bomb might cause less damage. [40]

Militarisation, however, was successful in achieving the goals laid down by Dame Katherine Jones. Registered nurses were afforded commissioned officer status in 1941 and this status was extended outwards from the army to include all nurses within the Royal Air Force, Royal Navy and Commonwealth nurses. Once hostilities had ceased, army nurses were established as a distinct corps and even managed to negotiate a 'professional' salary lead over members of the women's services. From being an ambiguous nursing unit they had established a firm place 'in and of the Army', though Dame Katherine's efforts were not appreciated by all nurses. Commonwealth nurses, for instance, resented the officer commissions and viewed them as an unwelcome military imposition on their 'civilian' vocation. There were also debates within the British services as to the value of militarisation. The Air Force in particular refused to align nurses with service pay, stating that pay should conform to the civilian Rushcliffe scales, and refused to give nurses military titles.[41]

The front line policy provided yet another focus for debate, this time between the British and Commonwealth forces. Military policy was inconsistent with regard to the deployment of women in operational areas. Confused evacuation procedures, which were initiated during a variety of campaigns, served to highlight this inconsistency. During the Greek campaign, for instance, British medical services decided that nurses should hold their position on the front line and risk capture, whereas Australian medical services insisted that nurses should be evacuated. Nurses themselves were eager to administer care on the front line where they believed their skills would be valued. Military officers generally supported this decision to work in operational areas because having a few pretty faces around was considered to be good for the morale of the troops,[42] although there were criticisms of the masculine style khaki uniform. Dame Katherine justified this change in uniform style on the grounds that khaki was more suitable for administering care in jungles and deserts and that it provided an important symbol of the front line policy. The Matron in Chief declared that:

> *Florence Nightingale, if she were alive now, would rejoice in the significance of this unfeminine apparel, for it means that we are getting ever closer to the front line.* [43]

There may have been some consternation within military circles with regard to Dame Katherine's policy but in the civilian nursing sector the changes were observed with glee. As the nursing press proclaimed:

The new khaki uniform which emphasises the military rank of members of QAIMNS is very impressive and becoming. [44]

Numerous articles explained the significance of officer status for registered nurses and highlighted the advantages of adapting the army pattern for the whole profession. It can also be argued that, since many nurses at this time were trained in the civilian sector in preparation for military service, the assimilation of military and civilian nursing in terms of rank was viewed as an ongoing and expedient process. [45]

Extending the Policy

Militarisation was accepted with varying degrees of enthusiasm by service nurses and, since the policy was a 'top down' initiative, it is difficult to assess the views of nurses working at ground level. Some clearly objected to military discipline and the extreme regimentation of nursing practice, while others supported these features in the interests of efficiency. In the civilian sector, however, militarisation became distorted. Nurse discipline became more severe and stressed the importance of class distinction, duty and self-sacrifice although, even during the inter-war period, punishment tasks were assigned to nurses who failed to comply with petty restrictions. In terms of nurse discipline, therefore, militarisation merely served to reinforce existing authoritarian regimes. In order to avoid these punishment tasks, the *Nursing Illustrated* advised nurses to use 'the application of intelligent acquiescence' when dealing with superiors. [46]

Further manifestations of militarisation included racism, the introduction of military style ward inspections and ceremonial functions that included the presentation of 'medals'. In addition, nurses' uniforms were 'crossed with a strain of militarism, often to denote rank' [47] and incorporated a 'mess dress'. In their eagerness to identify with concepts of military efficiency, nurses adopted an obsessive manner towards the punctuality of ward routines and a military attitude towards personal appearance. Nurses' shoes were expected to gleam, shoulder epaulettes had to be aligned with creases on sleeves, plus aprons were overly starched. Daily appraisals by the matron ensured that nurses were assessed much like soldiers on parade. However, despite this enthusiasm to identify with military efficiency, the concept itself was largely a myth. The forces were nowhere near as efficient in practice as they were perceived to be in theory. Their efficient images were maintained by glossing over incidents of bungling and, in order to assimilate with the military pattern, civilian nurses did likewise. Even if nurses were lacking in competence they were instructed to assume an air of confidence. This process of bluff was also used to reassure patients in times of medical crisis.

Although patients appeared to be blissfully unaware of nursing incompetence, they were nonetheless made painfully aware of the militarisation of nursing practice[48] since identification with masculinity had permeated the sphere of patient care. Nurse character traits that were associated with femininity, such as the expression of sympathy, tenderness and compassion, were systematically discouraged, whereas a brisk functional 'masculine' approach towards patient care was actively endorsed. Thus the traditional image of the nurse was transformed from that of an 'angel of mercy' to that of an unfeeling 'battleaxe'. Much of this shift in gender identity reflected a wider wartime trend, as women recognised that anything associated with the military and masculinity was afforded higher status and access to power than anything associated with femininity.[49] The gender shift in nursing was accelerated by the profession's urgent desire to shed the image of motherhood, and the masculine approach towards patient care was designed to portray nursing skills in a more professional light. Identification with the military provided further prestige both in terms of masculinity and social class. Therefore, as far as registered nurses were concerned, their status was significantly elevated once they were equated with the military 'officer class'.

Interpretations of the 'officer class', however, varied within the profession. For most registered nurses, officer status merely confirmed their membership of an elite social class and endorsed their legitimate authority over less qualified nurses. Others adopted a broader interpretation of the term and argued that 'officer' nurses should ideally possess similar character traits to those normally required for military leadership. This broader interpretation of the 'officer class' nurse formed the basis of the Horder Reports of 1942, 1943 and 1949. The Royal College of Nursing had established a 'Nursing Reconstruction Committee' chaired by Lord Horder in 1941 and subsequent reports provided by Horder stressed that 'officer class' nurses were essential in order to stimulate professional development. According to Horder, the main function of the officer class nurse was to provide professional leadership. Unfortunately, it was precisely this aspect of 'officer' status that the majority of nurses failed to grasp. This failure highlighted a fundamental civilian distortion of the military nursing model and, in the long term, served to impede the course of professional development.

Status Reviewed

Although nurses had failed to grasp the realities of the military officer role, they had adopted the symbolic trappings of military organisation. Such enthusiastic identification with military ideology was designed to elevate nurse status and aid recruitment, but how successful was this strategy in achieving these goals? Military style cadet schemes, for instance, certainly helped to resolve staff shortages. However, the fact that cadets were allowed to perform skilled nursing tasks ultimately undermined the position of the registered nurse and placed the patient at the mercy of untrained fifteen-year-old girls. There was also an alternative potential labour force which was never fully exploited. According to correspondence in the nursing and national press, many older women would have been prepared to undertake nurse training, but probationer nurses were required to be under thirty-five years of age to enter training. Matrons generally preferred to employ young girls as they made for a more compliant workforce. Furthermore, despite the lifting of the marriage bar, restrictions such as compulsory residence in nurses' homes precluded the employment of married nurses.

The way in which nurses were treated by their superiors also deterred many women from returning to the profession. As Lord Crook discovered when investigating claims of unnecessary nurse discipline, there were many instances where petty restrictions had impinged on the social lives of nurses. He informed the House of Lords that:

> *In one of the cases I investigated recently, a married woman who had gone back in widowhood to her original profession of nursing left the ward at eight o'clock and went to the local cinema, where the main film started at 8.40pm and finished at about 9.50pm. She decided to stop to the end and, as a result, arrived back at the nurses' home at ten minutes past ten. She was made to stand outside the door of the night sister for fifteen to twenty minutes and reprimanded like a child.* [50]

This incident was typical of thousands more which occurred on a regular basis across the country. Occasionally, more liberal matrons attempted to ease the restrictions, particularly with respect to student nurses, but their efforts were usually met with widespread dissension:

> *One young matron, seeing the absurdity of this ten o'clock rule, prepared to have keys cut which could be distributed to nurses to allow them to come into the home after a social engagement. The*

> *nurses who received the keys were very happy but the sisters of the*
> *wards resigned the following morning as a protest against the*
> *lack of discipline shown by the matron.* [51]

There was no evidence to suggest that discipline was less harsh in the military nursing sector than in the civilian field yet, in stark contrast to the civilian nursing services, the military nursing services were flooded with applications from women eager to join their ranks. As Baly has argued, the elitist image and attractive uniform contributed to the popularity of service nursing.[52] But to view this popularity merely in terms of uniform and elitism negates more fundamental issues. Since territorial reserve and conscript nurses were not allowed to wear the distinctive red capes associated with the QA nursing unit, the uniform was not necessarily responsible for attracting recruits, besides which the QA uniform was changed to a far less distinctive khaki during the war. Evidently the elitism of military nursing provided a greater recruitment incentive, particularly since the demands of war had eroded civilian nurse status, but nurses were also attracted to military service by the very same features which attracted their male colleagues.

As Summers has argued:

> *Military nursing gave respectable expression to less admissible*
> *female emotions. To be a nurse in war was to be abroad, free of*
> *domestic ties and comforts, ready to surmount hardship and*
> *encounter danger. It could bring a woman to the heart of the*
> *action on a world stage.* [53]

Although this statement was made in relation to the Boer War and the First World War, it was no less accurate when applied to the Second World War. Hatred of the enemy was not given as an expressed reason for enlisting, and nurses were drawn to the military by the prospect of danger, excitement and wanting to be in the thick of things. The elitism associated with military nursing undoubtedly boosted recruitment figures, but for most nurses the primary appeal of the military rested on the opportunities that accompanied enlistment. In terms of recruitment, civilian nursing could not hope to compete with a service that offered women an opportunity to participate in an international war experience.

Therefore, despite the fact that between February 1943 and September 1946 'some £166,000 was spent out of public funds on nursing publicity',[54] civilian recruitment campaigns achieved very little, although, given the appeal of the forces, it was not surprising that propaganda emphasised the connections between military and civilian nursing. However, it can be argued that authoritarian regimes in the civilian sector did more to deter nurse recruitment than encourage it, neither did these same regimes appear to raise nurse status unless, as some women argued, there was a certain status attached to being a martyr to the cause. Many nurses believed that identification with the military 'officer class' did provide a certain prestige; this belief was underpinned by the prevailing attitudes of the medical profession.

Sir Robert Hutchinson, consultant at the Royal London Hospital, for instance, claimed that 'Royal London nurses were like the Brigade of Guards, the pick of the Forces'. Sir Robert also praised the obedience of nurses and reiterated the neofeudalist stance on education, stating that 'a nurse's character is far more important than brains'.[55] Unquestioning obedience could not possibly be equated with notions of professionalism but, as far as nurses were concerned, militarism could be equated with elevated status. Alhough a status which was based on a hierarchical structure of social and racial injustice, combined with obsessive ideas of perceived efficiency, was unlikely to afford any long-term professional security. It can also be argued that as the profession became increasingly 'masculinised', the traditional 'feminine' nurturing qualities associated with nursing were ultimately devalued.

Conclusion

The nursing profession emerged from the Second World War ill-prepared for any form of reconstruction. Civilian nurses were politically fragmented and weakened by a diminished ratio of trained to untrained staff, whereas military nurses were better organised and, in terms of recruitment, had prepared for the post-war competition which came in the form of the newly established women's services. Government policy with regard to nurses continued to concentrate on improving recruitment levels since there was no doubt that civilian healthcare delivery had suffered as a result of wartime nursing shortages.

Throughout the early stages of the war, organisation of the nursing services was minimal and ineffective. In terms of exerting control on the profession as a whole, 1943 was the year of action. The Nurses Act, Rushcliffe recommendations, civilian nurse conscription, the VAD Committee and restrictions on military nurse conscription were all policy initiatives implemented in the same year. These policies formed the basis of nurse organisation from 1943 onwards and represented, with the addition of the direction of labour plan in 1944, maximum state control over nurse organisation. When applied to the complex issues that surrounded nursing shortages, however, maximum control proved to be almost as ineffective as the minimalist approach.

The 'carrot and stick' policy adopted by government officials had failed to improve the situation. The explanations for this failure were threefold: firstly, by the time Rushcliffe pay scales were introduced, the rise in the cost of living had largely negated the effects of salary improvements; secondly, because nurses had exploited the training exemption in the Control of Engagement Order, only the midwifery sector had gained from direct controls; and finally, the introduction of the Nurses Act had served to alienate large sections of the nursing workforce by undermining nurse status and reducing professional autonomy.

In fairness to government policy makers, it was difficult to maintain a balance between the number of nurses needed for the fighting forces and those required for civilian healthcare delivery. They were unable to predict the course of the war and adjust the situation accordingly. However, difficulties such as those associated with the Civil Nursing Reserve were predictable. A more rational assessment of the nursing labour force conducted during the early stages of war, together with an overall strategy for dealing with potential problems, may have produced a more efficient and cohesive nursing force.

The nursing appointments at the Ministry of Health, Ministry of Labour and the Colonial Office clearly had some impact on policy formulation since nurse organisation began to improve slightly from 1941 onwards. However, status issues continued to dominate professional thinking and the militarisation policy pursued by Dame Katherine Jones was indicative of this concern. As she herself proclaimed:

> *If I survive at all in nursing history I shall doubtless survive as the militarising Matron in Chief. I am glad that it should be so. I have in fact done my best to militarise QAIMNS and the TANS but I should like as many people as possible to know why I have done this and to realise that there is method in my madness.* [56]

Despite Dame Katherine's 'method and madness', it can be argued that militarisation prevailed in the civilian sector primarily because professionalisation had failed. Within the military itself, the policy achieved specific goals. Military nurses had secured their place within the service framework. They became a corps in the post-war years and, for the most part, chose to train their own nurses rather than merely accept those who had been trained in civilian hospitals. They had also gained financial ground over their civilian counterparts.[57] The Ministry of Health acknowledged that higher salaries were justified for military nurses because of their position as officers in the armed forces. In addition to this monetary reward, officer status also gave military nurses a degree of political leverage within the services.

Within the civilian sector, nurses had no such political leverage. As the NHS emerged, nurses were rapidly swallowed up by a growing number of other healthcare professionals. Furthermore, when Dame Katherine Jones had advocated the imposition of a military framework on civilian nursing, the possible effects of this imposition on patient care had not been anticipated. That civilian nursing practice needed to diverge from that of the military became increasingly apparent in the post-war years.

However, the technological changes that had occurred within the military from 1939 onwards had exposed the weaknesses of 'aristocratic militarism' since technology demanded intellectual knowledge. Consequently, military training and nursing shifted in the direction of education and professionalism. Civilian nursing did not experience a similar shift in direction. War had accelerated medical research but technical advances in areas such as blood transfusions, radiography, physiotherapy and antibiotic therapy were initially slow to infiltrate civilian hospitals and communities. Although medical technology eventually revealed the inadequacies of nurse education, the profession chose to defend the practical system of nurse training. This resistance to reform had extensive ramifications for civilian post-war nursing.

Clearly, nurses failed to fight militarism from 1939 onwards. Instead, they openly advocated military identification in the vain hope that, once registered nurse status was linked to military officer class status, the overall position of the professional nurse would improve. This endorsement of militarism proved to be misguided since it acted as an immovable obstacle to change. Nurses were drawn to military ideology initially to secure state registration and continued to endorse it in an effort to raise and protect this status. Subsequently, civilian nurses were encumbered by an anti-educational bias and an outmoded system of discipline, combined with a paramilitary organisational structure that precluded any flexibility of nursing practice.

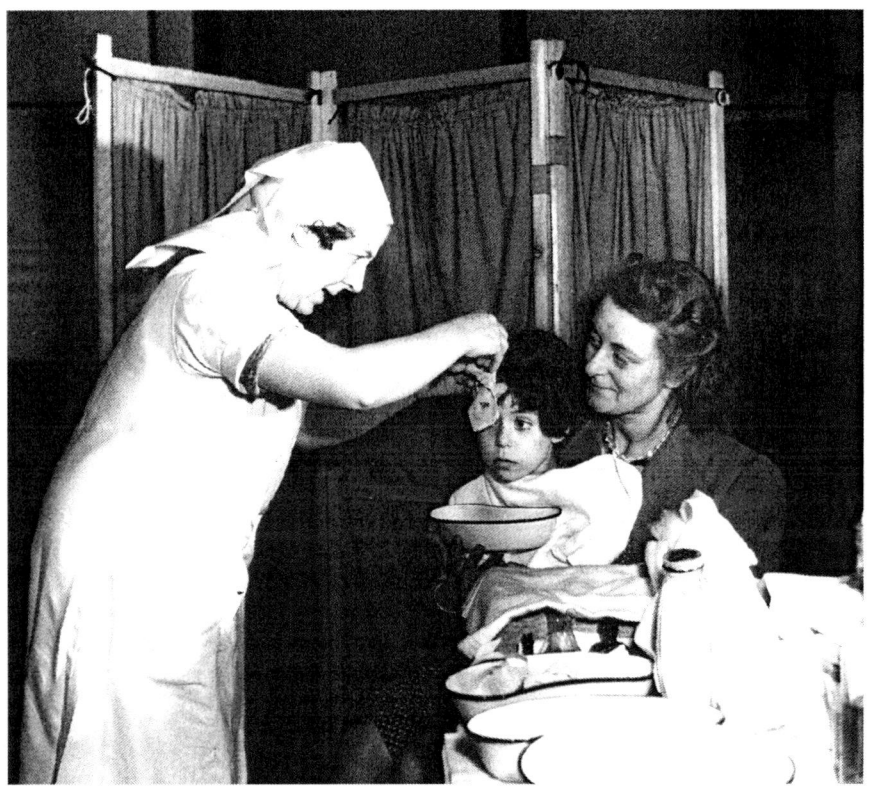

1944 Rest Centre - A nurse attends to a slight head wound caused by flying glass to a six year old girl whose home has been badly damaged by the blast.

Endnotes

(1)   By April 1940, Bartholomews Hospital, one of the largest in London, had only 145 beds available for civilian patients out of a bed total of 780. While the situation was less severe in rural areas, the ratio of bed allocation for civilians posed problems in several major cities.

(2)   The manner in which the British government organised medical and nursing procedures during the Second World War was influenced to some extent by experience gained by Spanish medical personnel during the Spanish Civil War. Barcelona had been subjected to over 340 air raids and the treatment of Spanish casualties had revolutionised medical opinion in Britain.

(3)   Athlone was disbanded in war but Committee findings were resurrected by Rushcliffe in 1943.

(4)   For example, female nurses assumed responsibility for operating theatres for the first time during the Second World War. It was also the first time female nurses were allowed to work in India.

(5)   *Parliamentary Debates* (House of Commons), 5th ser., 372, 13th June 1940, col.1456. Debate between members of the Supply Committee and the Ministry of Health, War Services.

(6)   'Hospital emergency schemes' *Nursing Illustrated*, 25th August 1939, p.2

(7)   The VAD scheme was first introduced in 1909 as a result of an Army Council initiative.

(8)   For background on Association of Hospital Matrons, see Abel-Smith, *op cit.*

(9)   The 'phony war' is usually interpreted as the period between 3rd September 1939 and the start of the Norwegian campaign on 9th April 1940.

(10)   Registered nurses had undergone a three-year training period leading to state registration whereas assistant nurses had some nursing experience but were not registered. Auxiliaries in the Civil Nursing Reserve were frequently women with no previous nursing experience.

(11)   IWM, 536/172/K9584, Report of Committee on Voluntary Aid Detachments, 1943.

(12)   P.G. Cambray and G.G.B. Briggs, *Official History of Red Cross and St John* (1949), p.664

(13)   Report of Committee on VADs, *op cit.*

(14)   RCNA RCN/C143/3, oral history transcript.

(15)   P. Summerfield, *Women Workers in the Second World War* (1989), p.74

(16)   *Ibid.*

(17)   S. Encel, 'The Study of Militarism in Australia', in J. van Doorn, ed. *Armed Forces and Society: sociological* essays (The Hague, 1968), p.138

(18)   Civilian cadets were taught subjects such as needlework and many refused to attend college on the grounds that lecturers rarely turned up. Others could not afford the bus fares to colleges.

(19)   Cambray and Briggs, *op. cit.*, p.415

(20)   *Ibid.*, p.416

(21)   *Ibid.*, p.415

(22)   *British Nursing Journal*, May 1945, editorial.

(23)   M. Baly, *Nursing and Social Change* (1980), p.172

(24)   Figures kept by the GNC were not totally reliable since many nurses on the register were not practising and some had died years earlier!

(25)   IWM K9775, p.6. Restrictions were imposed as a result of long discussions between Ministry of Health, Ministry of Labour and the War Office.

(26)   Baly, *op cit.*, p.173

(27)   PRO WO/222/178. Address to the East Anglian Group of the Association of Hospital Matrons by Dame Katherine Jones given on 2nd September 1944.

(28)   S. Bingham, *Ministering Angels* (1979), p.197

(29)   Edith Cavell originally trained at the Royal London Hospital and nursed during the First World War. She was held captive by Germans in Belgium and later shot to death.

(30)   *The Lamp still Burns* was released in 1943 and made with the co-operation and guidance of the Ministry of Health and, particularly, the senior nurses working at Whitehall at this time. The film emphasised the heroic nature of nursing in war, but also highlighted the discipline problems that deterred recruitment and prevented many nurses from continuing in the profession. Matrons came under attack for implementing the whole system of petty restrictions that were imposed on nurses both inside and outside their working hours. The film was seen as controversial by members of the profession and disturbing by members of the public. Nevertheless, it is perhaps the most accurate portrayal of civilian hospital nursing in Britain during the 1940s.

(31)   IWM 536/172/K9540. Government recruitment poster.
(32)   Dame Katherine Jones spent a total of 27 years as a nurse in the army and retired in 1944. Her militarisation policy began to emerge when she was mobilised on 11th September 1939 as Senior Principal Matron on the staff of the General Headquarters of the British Expeditionary Force.
(33)   A. Summers, *Angels and Citizens* (1988), p.28
(34)   Female units other than nursing were disbanded in 1918 because the War Office subscribed to the 'ten year' rule, i.e. war unlikely for ten years and women not needed.
(35)   PRO WO/222/178. Address to the East Anglian Group of the Association of Hospital Matrons by Dame Katherine Jones, given on 2nd September 1944. The AHM was founded in 1907 and organised on a regional basis to keep abreast of nursing developments around the country. The AHM, however, was not a progressive body.
(36)   *Ibid.*
(37)   J. Bassett, *Guns and Brooches* (Sydney 1992), p.121
(38)   *Royal London Hospital Nurses League Review*, XI (1942). This particular nurse died in action.
(39)   PRO WO/222/189/10. Extracts from the letters of military nurses.
(40)   *Ibid.*
(41)   This stance by the RAF formed part of an ongoing trend. As the youngest service, the RAF was less entrenched in military tradition and often challenged War Office policy. Subsequently, RAF nurses did not fully align with the other services until 1953.
(42)   In particular, nurses received support for their front line policy from Lord Mountbatten and Field Marshall Montgomery.
(43)   PRO WO/222/178. Address to the East Anglian group of the AHM by Dame Katherine Jones, 2nd September 1944.
(44)   *British Nursing Journal*, January 1945, p.3
(45)   Until army nurses were established as a corps, registered nurses were trained only in the civilian sector.
(46)   *Nursing Illustrated*, 1st September 1939, p.885
(47)   Baly, *op cit.*, p.213
(48)   This issue is examined in greater depth in Chapter 8.
(49)   C. Hooper, Manly States: Masculinities, International Relations & Gender Politics (New York Columbia Press, forthcoming December 2,000)
(50)   *Parliamentary Debates* (House of Lords), 5th ser., 159, 9th November 1948, p.290
(51)   *Ibid.*
(52)   Baly, *op cit.*, p.187 : The elitism of military nursing units centred on the notion of 'class' superiority. Military nurses were recruited primarily from the ranks of officers' wives, widows and daughters. The elitist image of these units was further underpinned by royal patronage.
(53)   Summers, *op cit.*, p.2
(54)   PRO MH/55/2074
(55)   *Royal London Hospital Nurses League Review*, XV (1946), p.11
(56)   PRO WO/222/178. Dame Katherine Jones, 2nd September 1944
(57)   Military nurses protected their status by refusing to take on 'regulars' for the duration of war and were far outnumbered by reservists. By 1945 the QAIMNS had expanded from 624 to 12,000, the QARNNS from 78 to 1,341 and the PMRAFNS from 171 to 1,215.

Chapter 3

Revolution or Evolution?
The Issue of Nursing Reform

Although the 1944 Government White Paper outlined a strategy for healthcare delivery within a National Health Service (NHS), it contained only a brief reference to the nursing services. Government officials were involved in 'medical and political horse-trading surrounding the establishment of the NHS'[1] and nursing services were relegated to a secondary position. Defects within the existing system of nursing organisation, particularly training and education, had been identified by a government working party chaired by Sir Robert Wood. But other than ensuring that nurses were recruited and trained in adequate numbers to staff the Health Service, there was no discernible government policy regarding the nursing profession. The General Nursing Council (GNC) for their part were, as Clay observed, 'anxious to preserve the system, nervous of radical change and determined to move only as far as they were pushed'.[2] The Wood Report had concluded in 1947 that nurse education needed to be separated from the service demands of hospitals and advocated radical changes. These included full student status and a reduction in the training period for registration, the abolition of assistant nurses and the introduction of a training scheme for orderlies. Wood's proposals were designed to increase the educational content of nurse training in order to provide a more flexible nursing service. Unfortunately, these proposals were rejected by the nursing establishment, which insisted that nursing should be rooted in a practical training scheme that exuded an anti-educational bias throughout.

Albeit inconsistent with the rejection of reform, attempts to reintroduce the minimum educational level formed the basis of GNC policy during the post-war years. The GNC argued that a minimum educational level was necessary to improve professional status. The government, meanwhile, resisted these attempts until 1962 as they feared that such a policy would adversely affect recruitment. Throughout this period, according to White, 'nursing was dominated by the Ministry of Health',[3] and the premise for this assumption appears to hinge on the fact that the GNC were required to gain Ministry approval before making any adjustments to nurse training courses. However, senior nurses at the Ministry of Health were also required to seek GNC approval before they were able to initiate changes. The argument expressed by White, therefore, has ignored this two-way process and negated the influence exerted by the GNC and other professional organisations. It should also be recognised that neither the government nor the nursing profession acted as a unified body with regard to policy formulation and implementation and national policy was often at variance with local policy. In addition, the confused dynamics of the decision-making process itself further obscured the relationship between government and nursing policy.

Radical changes in nursing organisation should have accompanied the radical changes in healthcare delivery. But as the NHS evolved, the government continued to view policy initiatives only in the light of how they would affect nurse recruitment. The nursing establishment were equally blinkered; all policy was considered in the light of how nurse status would be affected. It was not until the mid 1950s that the blinkers were removed on both sides. Government officials switched their attention and concentration onto the administrative structure of nursing. The GNC, prompted by technical changes in medical and nursing practice, tentatively shifted policy direction towards education and research.

In view of the time span which was allowed to elapse between the identification of problems and policy initiatives designed to combat them, obstacles to change are worthy of further examination. Why did gradualism succeed in place of radical reform measures? The shortcomings within the existing system of nurse organisation were clearly visible in 1945, so why were nurses so anxious to preserve the system? As reports had already suggested that the system was responsible for alienating potential nurse recruits, why did the government fail to initiate reform? It is possible that the answers to these questions can be found by examining the existence of a military imposition on civilian nursing organisation, the extent of which was never fully understood either by the participants within the nursing profession or those outside it. As a result of the Second World War, society generally had been militarised. As Cooter has observed, not only were 'military values and attitudes carried into civilian spheres' but, more fundamentally, society and economics were coming to be disciplined in accordance with military conceptions of efficiency.[4] Military influence within civilian nursing realms was arguably considered both normal and desirable. In terms of recruiting and training personnel there was a general assumption that the armed forces had found a 'magic formula'. Moreover, it was further believed that this formula provided an example for the rest of society, a view expounded by Wood and Cohen in their reports of 1947 and 1948. Faced with a seemingly intractable nurse recruitment problem and high student wastage rates, the Ministry of Health and the Ministry of Labour were eager to learn this formula. Albeit for different reasons, therefore, both government and nursing camps identified with military ideology.

The government, however, whilst not averse to change, had no desire to initiate major nursing reform. Having created a division of nursing at the Ministry of Health during the war and having prepared the groundwork with the Wood Report, government officials believed that the profession would introduce change. The fact that nurses failed to seize the initiative led to some confusion at ministerial level and, as Clay has commented, 'In the history of missed opportunities, surely the fate of the Wood Report deserves a chapter of its own'.[5] Resistance to change encompassed all areas of nursing development and practice and government officials initially underestimated the strength of this resistance. The pervading military ethos within the GNC, along with sections of the RCN and the Association of Hospital Matrons (AHM), constituted the main obstacle to change. As Dame Elizabeth Cockayne had noted in her term as Chief Nursing Officer at the Ministry of Health, together these bodies 'formed a group within the profession and it was difficult to stand outside it. They were all committee people and conservative with a small "c"'.[6]

Over a period of time, however, the government appeared to recognise the negative influence exerted on the profession by the GNC. Consequently, a curious scenario developed whereby, as far as possible, the GNC was excluded from the policy-making process. Rather than adopt a confrontational approach towards the GNC, the government attempted to bypass the problem. In order to fully comprehend this situation this chapter will examine the role of the GNC and the reactions of both government and nursing camps to the prospect of reform.

Resistance to Reform: Views from Outside the Ranks

Ideally, the reform measures outlined by the Wood Report in 1947 should have been incorporated into the 1949 Nurses Act. The implementation of such reforms would have resulted in a more flexible nursing service, able to respond to changing healthcare demands. However, in place of reform the nursing profession adhered rigidly to its own body of traditions 'which were drawn from the army, from religious orders and possibly from the new girls' public schools'.[7] Subsequently, various arguments have been formulated in an attempt to explain why nurses rejected reform and, consequently, why the 1949 Act 'failed significantly to achieve any reconstruction'.[8]

Abel-Smith, for instance, has argued that 'there was no support from the leaders of the profession for the more radical proposals of the Wood Committee'.[9]

While Dingwall *et al* have argued that the nursing profession appeared 'almost Luddite in their opposition to a strengthening of the educational aspects of training',[10] White on the other hand has pointed out that GNC objections to Wood centred on the genuine reservations that a reduced training period would downgrade nurse status, while Baly has maintained that the publication of a minority report by Dr Cohen, which advocated the need for further research, reduced the overall impact of Wood. However, before discussing the validity of these arguments it is necessary to examine the role of the GNC and the contents of both the Wood and Cohen reports. Why did the publication of these reports serve to alienate the nursing profession? How were potential reforms viewed in government and nursing circles? More importantly, why was gradualism allowed to triumph in place of radical reform?

According to Dame Elizabeth Cockayne, CNO at the Ministry of Health in 1948, the GNC as the statutory body controlling nurse education and training 'did not welcome views from outside their ranks'.[11] However, from 1932 onwards the nursing profession was increasingly subjected to views and reports initiated from 'outside the ranks'. Not surprisingly, the GNC adopted a defensive position. Having gained statutory authority to organise nurse training and registration in 1919, they had struggled to ensure that training schools maintained an acceptable standard, frequently in the face of government opposition. Government reports relating to nurse training, therefore, were regarded with deep suspicion. The GNC believed that government ministers were totally ignorant of nursing affairs.

However, as a result of the Second World War, senior nurses were appointed in an advisory capacity at the Ministry of Health and the Ministry of Labour and, consequently, the government could no longer be accused of being ignorant of nursing issues. Furthermore, these same senior nurses were involved in compiling the government-initiated Wood report and desperately wanted nursing reform. Unfortunately, these nurses were in the minority and, as Dame Elizabeth recalled, 'the Matron's Association never forgave her for the report'.[12] Nursing reaction to the Wood proposals had exposed a crisis in terms of professional leadership. Traditionally, members of the GNC and senior nurses of the RCN together represented nursing leadership, but the creation of a nursing division at the Ministry of Health had challenged this position. Furthermore, while the GNC were anxious to preserve the system, nurses at Whitehall were equally anxious to change it.

The government was unaware of the rift that existed between the levels of nurse leadership. The Wood Committee were advised in 1946 that:

> *... the impending establishment of a National Health Service*
> *would undoubtedly increase the demand for nurses even above*
> *the present level, and thus rendered a comprehensive review of*
> *the whole nursing service and its problems of first importance.* [13]

Since nurses were involved with the Committee in compiling the research for
the Wood report and in formulating the proposals for an alternative training
scheme, the government assumed that such proposals would find favour with
the profession generally. Nurses at the Ministry of Health and the Ministry of
Labour were dynamic and innovative. In this respect, however, they were also
unusual.

Senior nurses involved with the GNC and the RCN tended to be representative
of the older generation of nurses. They firmly believed that the removal of
domestic work, long hours and repetitive tasks from nurse training would, in
effect, deprive 'the student nurse not only of the ability to nurse but of
satisfaction in nursing'.[14] This belief reflected the neofeudalist stance towards
education traditionally associated with the aristocratic military model since,
within the army, the criterion of 'intellect' was traditionally associated with
general incompetence.[15] GNC policy therefore continued to be dominated by
the view that character was more important than intellect and that nurses were
'born not made'. Wood had attempted to counteract this view by asserting that
although 'common sense and good judgement' were indispensable nursing
characteristics, they did not form 'a complete equipment for attacking social
problems'.[16]

While the Wood Report aimed to assess the potential nursing requirements of
the NHS, its actual findings shocked the nursing profession. As the report
stated:

> *In the course of studying the work of 36 student nurses our*
> *investigators came across no instance of any formal teaching in*
> *the wards. A student nurse, even after many weeks in a ward, may*
> *know neither the names of the patients nor the ailments from*
> *which they suffer.* [17]

The report also examined in detail the causes of student wastage and declared
that:

> *... the conclusion emerges clearly from this analysis that the type*
> *of discipline which pervades the training schools today is*

unquestionably the most important cause of wastage. This code of discipline is intelligible historically inasmuch as it was originally inspired by a conventional tradition. [18]

Remaining causes of wastage were attributed to the attitudes of senior nurses towards senior staff and, to a lesser extent, the poor quality of food, long hours and pressure of work.

Members of the Wood Committee believed that a realistic approach was needed to resolve wastage problems, as revealed by the following statement:

Experience teaches that, as far as the first two causes are concerned, it is of little use merely appealing to hospital authorities to modify discipline or to adopt more understanding attitudes. The introduction of structural changes in the organisation and staffing of training schools is certainly needed. [19]

Further recommendations included the introduction of selection tests, both for new recruits to the nursing profession and for registered nurses applying for senior nursing positions. These personality tests, designed by military psychologists, would, it was argued, ensure that new recruits were in fact suitable to undertake nursing and that those working to obtain senior nursing positions were capable of fostering good relationships with junior staff. Recent experience gained in military realms had, according to Wood, confirmed the 'worth of mental tests in effective selection for training'. [20]

Nurses were submitted to mental tests as part of the working party field study and analysis of test results revealed that student nurses were, on average, more intelligent than trained nurses. The Committee concluded that this was perhaps because more able students were leaving the profession before qualifying. Nurses were apparently more intelligent than the general population, although it was realised that the Matrix was more effective in predicting levels of intelligence at the upper end of the scale rather than at the lower end.

The population statistics were based on:

... the standardisation of Matrix results employed by the Army. The mean Matrix score in a representative sample of 5,000 men in the Army is 34.4, with S.D. = 9.8; the mean Matrix score of a standard group of 3,759 seamen in the Royal Navy is 36.9,

S.D. = 7.4. The estimated mean score of all hospital nurses is 36.6, S.D. = 9.5.[21]

Data further confirmed that, in many instances, assistant nurses were equally as intelligent as their registered counterparts. Moreover, around 20% to 25% of hospital trained nurses would be capable of undertaking educational courses at university level. These were the nurses who achieved a Matrix score of 46 and above and who were comparable with university-educated men serving in the Army who were subjected to the same tests.

While intelligence tests were advocated by Wood for potential nursing recruits, the report also stressed the need to use these in conjunction with personality selection tests. The methods used were described in the 'Expert Committee on the work of Psychologists and Psychiatrists in the Services'.[22] As previously acknowledged, nurses had identified with both the military and masculinity during the war years as a means of raising their professional status. Research studies which incorporated personality tests reflected this identification and supposedly proved that nurses were, in fact, more masculine by nature than other females. As Wood explained:

> *Practising nurses as judged by these tests, tended to achieve more 'masculine' scores than any other female occupational group except teachers in secondary schools and colleges. Practising nurses and domestic servants stood at two ends of the scale, the nurses at the masculine end and the domestic servants at the feminine end. This may explain why the attempt to burden student nurses with nursing and domestic tasks calling, apparently, for diametrically opposed qualities, breaks down in the form of wastage.* [23]

It was therefore concluded that nurses should be relieved of domestic duties in order to concentrate on the more masculine task of nursing! Relieving student nurses of their domestic duties could also reduce registration training to a period of eighteen months and specialist training could be provided in a period of six months. Wood recommended that area nurse training committees should be established to administer both registration and post-registration courses.

Given the overall content of the Wood Report, it was not surprising that it failed to endear itself to senior nurses. Firstly, by advocating full 'student status' for trainee nurses, the report directly challenged the pervading neofeudalist approach to nurse education. Secondly, the type of discipline exerted by senior nurses over junior staff was identified as the primary cause of student wastage. Thirdly, not only did the report conclude that many of these juniors were more intelligent than their seniors, but the proposed need for selection tests implied that matrons were unable to judge the suitability of nursing candidates. Finally, to add insult to injury, the report announced that the GNC were not:

> *... favourably placed to lay down and implement an educational policy for the nursing profession; they have very little educational representation and no counterpart to the academic representation on the General Medical Council.* [24]

Viewed in this light, GNC opposition to Wood was not merely a question of resistance to reform but rather a fight for its own survival as a statutory body responsible for nurse education.

The nursing profession was still recovering from the shock of the Wood report when a further blow was inflicted by the publication of a minority report in 1948. The report was compiled by Dr Cohen, who had been involved in the original investigations for the Wood analysis but had dissented from signing the majority report because a 'divergence of view existed'[25] between Dr Cohen and his colleagues. According to Dr Cohen, the original research findings regarding conditions in nurse training schools had been 'toned down' for the Wood report to avoid alienating the profession. This process of distorting the evidence was 'unscientific', as the minority report explained:

> *Scientific method, where applicable, must be followed wherever it leads and the unpalatability of relevant facts must not prevent them from being brought to light. For example, a toning down of nursing conditions in training schools, mental hospitals or public assistance institutions must be resisted, for the work of a social scientist, like that of his medical colleague, is nullified if he shirks the unpleasant aspects of the situation under study.* [26]

Far from shirking the unpleasant findings uncovered by research, Dr Cohen exposed them and argued that although more research was needed, nursing reforms should be implemented immediately. The minority report contained letters from individual nurses which revealed the reasons why many of them had abandoned the profession. The letters also described the extent to which nursing practice had succumbed to military style regimentation. The following extracts from nurses' letters, taken directly from the minority report, provide some insight into the nature of this militarisation process:

The reign of the Sergeant Major still continues in very many wards and only results in the frequent resignation of trained and untrained staff. I greatly objected to the lack of privacy in the nurses' homes. Cupboards and drawers were periodically inspected by the homes sister; letters were given out irregularly through a hatch because it was said that nurses could not be trusted to take their own.[27]

So many sisters set themselves up as demi-gods demanding blind obedience from their subordinates. The matron is often a person with a very primly starched cap and apron, who makes a daily inspection tour of the ward, while nurses stand with bated breath hoping she will not notice that the corner of number 26's bed is not quite straight.[28]

Surely after the long hours we work we are entitled to a little recreation in our private lives. Most of the rules are petty, such as no flowers allowed in bedrooms, no shoes on the floor, nothing on the window sills or dressing tables, nurses to be indoors by 10.30pm, lights out at 11pm. No-one to take a bath after 10pm. A round is done by the Home Sister to see that these rules are carried out.[29]

The hardest task of all - that is complying with all the petty restrictions, which in most cases are worse than the Armed Forces.[30]

Priority given to tidying of lockers and straightening of beds before the care of patients.[31]

Discipline developed into class distinction and obliteration of all feelings.[32]

Within my own experience I found that there is a general feeling of suppression, one feels like a mouse must feel when tormented by a cat and cannot get free.[33]

The senior staff needed to treat the junior staff as human beings and not as automatons. I have been in the Army as you see and though there is plenty of discipline and Red Tape there, there is still a more human element in it than I found in the hospital.[34]

> *Discipline was carried to an extreme, so much so that it was frightening and disturbing.*[35]

> *Life on the wards to me was one long nightmare. I did my best with work that was entirely new to me, only to be very severely reprimanded if anything was wrong, and usually in front of all the patients. Sister never tried to help us, she was just there trying to find fault.*[36]

However, while the Wood report had antagonised and shocked the nursing profession, Dr Cohen's minority report provoked extreme anger. *The British Nursing Journal* retaliated by publishing an open letter to Dr Cohen, asking:

> *Have you ever met a sharp tongued wife, Doctor? I have, and school mistresses, waitresses, shop assistants - butchers, bakers and candlestick makers. And for that matter, Doctor, we have all met many rude and sharp tongued members of your own Honourable profession.* [37]

Protests relating to the research findings of both Wood and Cohen continued to emanate from the nursing establishment. Dame Elizabeth was instrumental in compiling the Wood report and had tried to convince the GNC of its value. She recalled that 'with hindsight she feels that she could have used more "soothing language" but facts were facts'.[38] These same facts were debated intensely in the House of Commons and the House of Lords. As Lord Crook acknowledged, both 'the majority and minority reports ... make it very clear to all of us that the new health service has inherited a large quantity of very bad traditions and very bad conditions'. He also stressed that 'it is not true that pay is the fundamental difficulty of the nursing profession'.[39]

The government had, in fact, recognised that the fundamental problem within the profession centred on the need to separate nurse training from the provision of nursing services. Moreover, in response to the problem, the Minister of Health Aneurin Bevan drafted a Nurses Bill based on the Wood proposals. It is clear that Bevan demonstrated 'great goodwill towards nursing in the form taken by his draft proposals; they were sweeping and extraordinarily ambitious for a hitherto subsidiary occupation'.[40] An analysis of parliamentary debates throughout this period also reveals a wellspring of government support in favour of nursing reform. Indeed, many members of Parliament believed that major reform was to be the whole purpose of legislation. As one member stated during the third reading of the Nurses Bill, the 'crux of the bill is the separation of training from staffing'.[41] There were also indications that identification by registered nurses with the military 'officer class' had not gone unnoticed. During a debate that centred on the proposed title of Assistant Nurse, one MP enquired, 'Would not the honourable gentleman agree that state registered nurses should form the criterion of all kinds of nursing?' The gentleman replied, 'One might say the "aristocracy", but I would not necessarily say the "criterion"'.[42]

Although the initial drafting of the Nurses Bill was based on the Wood proposals, by the time the Bill had reached the statute books there was very little evidence of this fact. With the exception of area nurse training committees and some provision for experimentation in nurse education, the GNC and the RCN had ensured the rejection of Wood. The Nurses Act of 1949 amalgamated the male nurse register with the general register and closed supplementary sections. In effect, the Act was purely cosmetic. The GNC were empowered to introduce experimental training schemes, but were predictably reluctant to do so. The Area Nurse Training Committees were not established until 1951 and only a handful of university-linked courses existed:

> *The Act was a reflection of those changes which the nursing establishment (particularly the matrons) and the employers had permitted. It took no account of the critical recommendations made by post-war nursing reports.* [43]

The GNC had worked extremely hard to preserve the status quo and insisted that nurse training should remain within a practical domain. The government, believing that the implementation of reform would result in improved recruitment levels, had supported the Wood recommendations. There were also considerable financial reasons for doing so: 'The GNC line could be seen as unnecessarily costly, in that it committed the NHS to a large workforce with a modest level of education and a disproportionately long gap between entry and certification'.[44] The training system outlined by Wood, based on theoretical knowledge and the acquisition of specialist skills, allowed for greater flexibility in nursing practice. Nurse recruits trained within a period of eighteen months would be able to work unsupervised at an earlier stage, supported by a team of trained ward orderlies. The logic of these arguments, however, did not enter the equation as far as the GNC were concerned. Resistance to reform stemmed from entrenched cultural traditions and an overriding preoccupation with nurse status.

However, since the government favoured the implementation of nursing reform, why did ministers afford the GNC such political leverage? The GNC were denied permission to administer post-registration courses, but this denial represented the only real attempt on behalf of the government to oppose GNC demands. According to White, Bevan's refusal to allow the GNC any powers in relation to post-registration training was due to the fact that he had misunderstood Appendix VII of the Wood report. This appendix emphasised the need for post-registration courses in order to train specialist nurses. However, given that Bevan had discussed the Wood report at length with nursing advisers at the Ministry of Health, White's assumption that Bevan had misunderstood Appendix VII is highly questionable.[45]

In fact, Bevan's reluctance to extend GNC control in the area of nurse education demonstrated not only a clear understanding of both the Wood and Cohen reports, but also recognition of the GNC as the main obstacle to change. Furthermore, since the Wood report had stated that the GNC were not 'favourably placed' to formulate an educational policy for the nursing profession, there was no logical reason for the GNC to assume responsibility for post-registration training. Bevan had not, as White suggested, merely misunderstood an appendix in the Wood report; he had recognised the need for nurse specialism but doubted the suitability of the GNC to determine the educational content of specialist training. Bevan's steadfast position regarding this issue represented the first clear indication that government officials acknowledged the GNC as being 'more concerned with entry requirements than it was with nurse education itself'.[46]

The GNC never did manage to gain control of post-registration training and, as Dingwall *et al* have observed:

> *A hint of the Ministry's preference is provided by the separate provision under the Joint Board for Clinical Nursing Studies which was not placed under GNC control and which emphasised the provision of training in short, skill-specific modules throughout a nurse's career as the demands of the service changed.* [47]

The Joint Board of Clinical Nursing Studies was established by senior nurses at Whitehall through the Standing Nursing Advisory Committee, but it did not simply reflect ministerial preference. As Dame Kathleen Raven, Chief Nursing Officer (CNO) at the Ministry of Health from 1958 onwards, explained, policy changes were introduced through the Joint Board of Clinical Nursing Studies in order to make them 'acceptable to the profession'.[48] Senior nurses within the RCN had also attempted to improve the educational aspects of nurse training 'but always hit up against the GNC'.[49]

At one point during the tortuous passage of the Nurses Bill, 'the government appeared to be bracing itself to stand up to "that formidable body the General Nursing Council"'.[50] However, ministers eventually followed the path of least resistance. GNC educational influence was curtailed as far as possible and specialist training programmes were introduced through a 'back door' route. Why did ministers adopt this non-confrontational approach towards the GNC? The answer to this question lay with fundamental government policy - reform measures were evaluated primarily in relation to the issue of nurse recruitment; therefore, if the government considered reform to be an essential prerequisite for improving recruitment levels, then it was necessary for ministers to override GNC policy. However, in addition to outlining a new training scheme, Wood had provided valuable information aimed at resolving the difficulties associated with nurse recruitment. Ministers realised that it was possible to isolate this information and implement new recruitment strategies without the introduction of major reform. Confrontation with the GNC was thus avoided. As Dame Elizabeth recalled, ministers did not insist on nursing reform because they:

> ... had so much on their plates with all the other changes causing upheaval. The doctors had held up the inauguration of the National Health Service with their demands. There seemed to be no problem as regards money, but it was a mistake to think the Ministry could do everything. [51]

If the view which emerged from 'outside the ranks' of the nursing profession generally favoured reform, opinion 'inside the ranks' appeared to endorse the view adopted by the British Hospitals Association (BHA), which stated in 1948 that nurse training should be able:

> ... to produce a first class and sympathetic practical bedside nurse. To acquire her art and skill, the student in nursing must be as much apprentice as she is student. If she were to be given full student status, the trainee would acquire many grave misconceptions as to the nature of her professional life and her responsibilities as a practising nurse. [52]

Resisting the concept of Area Nurse Training Committees, the BHA announced that:

> *... the Association does not consider that the complete separation of nurse training, both in its control and finance, from that of the hospitals in which training must inevitably be done, 'desirable or practicable'.* [53]

The BHA continued its rhetoric by proclaiming that the plans outlined by Wood to establish Area Nurse Training Committees severely threatened the position and authority of the matron. This threat had not escaped the attention of the Association of Hospital Matrons (AHM), a group which echoed the views of the BHA and vehemently attacked the Wood proposals. Both the BHA and the AHM feared a loss of control over the nursing workforce and neither group appeared to consider potential reforms in terms of how they could improve healthcare delivery. While the Socialist Medical Association declared that reforms should be 'undertaken with the urgency that characterises a military operation',[54] there was no apparent sense of urgency within the nursing profession.

There were, however, some nurses who advocated change. As one senior nurse acknowledged in 1947, without reform 'there lies the danger that the profession may not always be organised for the greatest participation in and contribution to the health service of the people'.[55] Others, particularly those involved with the International Council of Nurses, recognised that it was primarily an entrenched attitude of mind which prevented progress. 'There was a division in the world as regards nursing, between those who followed Britain and those who followed America. The latter saw education as being much more important than the practical side.'[56] European states tended to follow the British nursing model since they shared similar aristocratic military traditions, whereas countries such as Australia and New Zealand veered towards the American model.

As a result of their military legacy, British nurses favoured the one aspect of the Wood report which they believed endorsed existing class distinctions. The proposed introduction of specialist university courses was welcomed by an anonymous group of nurse leaders called the 'Ten Group' as they argued that basic training 'could be regarded as experience in the ranks, a prerequisite for officer status'.[57] The Horder investigations, initiated by the RCN, also advocated the need for an 'officer class' nurse. Moreover, whereas Wood had suggested the abolition of the assistant nurse grade, Horder believed more assistants were required in order to gain 'more "other ranks" and relatively fewer "officer" nurses'.[58] Horder was severely critical of nurse training but approved of the overall hierarchical structure of nursing organisation. Degree courses were recommended, but only for 'officer class' nurses, and apprenticeship style courses for assistants. The Horder report largely reflected existing views within the profession and an analysis of the nursing press reveals that, for this reason, it did not provoke the same hostility as the Wood and Cohen publications. Although Horder had agreed with Wood regarding the need to separate nurse training from service demands, his report had not challenged the class basis and rank structure of the profession, or the role of the GNC. Over a decade later the situation was still unchanged and resistance to reform continued throughout the 1950s and 1960s.

The RCN initiated further investigations into the realms of nurse education in 1961 and the results were embodied in the Platt report of 1964. In most respects the report reiterated the Wood proposals. However, by suggesting that the implementation of new training schemes would inevitably necessitate changes in the structure and function of the GNC, Platt was doomed! For the most part, the GNC appeared to be preoccupied during the 1950s and 1960s with trying to identify the causes of student wastage, causes which had already been identified by Wood and Cohen. The GNC had responded to wastage problems by placing greater emphasis on military style selection procedures for new recruits. Traditional methods of nurse training and discipline were considered to be 'character forming' and therefore essential to 'nursing experience'. The character and background of nurse recruits took precedence over intellectual capabilities and the educational aspects of nurse training were continually relegated to a secondary position. The introduction of Area Nurse Training Committees in 1951 achieved little impact in relation to the overall structure of nurse training and the GNC did not strengthen the educational content of the general nurse training until 1969.[59]

The GNC had defended their position, arguing that it was not possible to strengthen educational aspects of nurse training without the introduction of the minimum educational requirement for entrants to the profession. In fairness to the GNC, a new syllabus was prepared to coincide with the introduction of the minimum educational level in 1962; its implementation, however, took considerably longer.[60] Neither did the GNC argument totally justify their position. The research findings published by Wood had already confirmed that student nurses were more intelligent than their superiors and were capable of undertaking degree courses. Furthermore, throughout this period, as Abel-Smith has demonstrated, 'not only had nursing been continuously recruiting better educated women' in relation to the population as a whole, 'it had also been obtaining an increasing proportion of such women'.[61] Moreover, many hospitals had demanded (and obtained) educational requirements from nurse recruits that exceeded the GNC recommended level. The GNC position, therefore, was indefensible and failure to expand the educational aspects of nurse training resulted in professional stagnation.

Conclusion

Clearly, nursing objections to the reforms outlined by Wood in 1947 did not dissipate with time, as witnessed by similar objections to the Platt recommendations of 1961. While Abel-Smith has suggested that nurse leaders were to blame for resisting reform, the validity of this view is dependent on the definition of nursing leadership. As previously acknowledged, nurse leaders in Whitehall agitated for reform. Obstacles to change did not therefore originate with nurse leaders such as Dame Elizabeth and Dame Kathleen but with the reluctance of nurses to follow such leadership. Alternatively, Baly has argued, change did not occur because Dr Cohen's Minority Report reduced the impact of Wood; yet Dr Cohen, while advocating the need for further research, also urged immediate reform. Indeed, his decision to dissent from signing the majority report rested, in part, on a divergence of opinion regarding the speed of reform. Introducing his minority report, Dr Cohen stated:

> *Nor can I sympathise with the view of the chairman, Sir Robert Wood, that 'at best the progress of reform is bound to be slow'. The rate of reform will rather depend on the will to act. The Services have shown what can be done where the will exists to initiate and swiftly execute vast new training projects. I see no reason for a less vigorous policy to be pursued in the sphere of health.* [62]

However, within civilian nursing realms two very different military models coexisted, giving rise to an ongoing tension between neofeudalist and techno-efficiency models of practice.

Clearly, the arguments expounded by Abel-Smith and Baly do not in themselves explain why the nursing profession objected to change. White's analysis, which maintains that GNC objections to reform centred on the belief that a reduced training period for nurses would result in reduced status, accurately reflects GNC considerations. The status argument, however, is connected with the 'Luddite' opposition to education noted by Dingwall *et al* and so it explains not only why nursing organisations resisted the Wood proposals but also why similar proposals outlined by Platt were rejected at a later date.

The fundamental problem, however, originated with nurses' perceptions of their status. Most nurses did not envisage a status linked to educational achievement but one that was rooted in military culture. Since nursing policy was primarily dictated by status concerns, the imposition of military values determined the scope and direction of nurse training. The anti-educational bias within the profession was a clear manifestation of long-standing military identification. Significantly, the only Wood recommendation adopted enthusiastically by the GNC was the introduction of selection tests for new recruits designed by military psychologists. These tests reaffirmed the GNC belief that it was the people entering the training system who were unsuitable rather than the system itself. The opportunity for educational reform was therefore lost because large sections of the nursing profession believed that nurses were 'born not made', a belief described by Asa Briggs as 'perhaps the most stubborn of all stereotypes'.[63] When the profession eventually shifted direction towards education and research, this did not always reflect a fundamental change in traditional beliefs. The shift was primarily motivated by technical advances in nursing and medical practice and the growing realisation that nurses required more theoretical education if the profession was to survive. The government, meanwhile, had expected nurses to implement reform and was surprised when they failed to seize the initiative. Ministers failed to intervene because major reform was not considered essential for improving nurse recruitment figures. The government therefore abandoned the GNC to its eternal debates regarding nurse status and concentrated on staffing the hospitals.

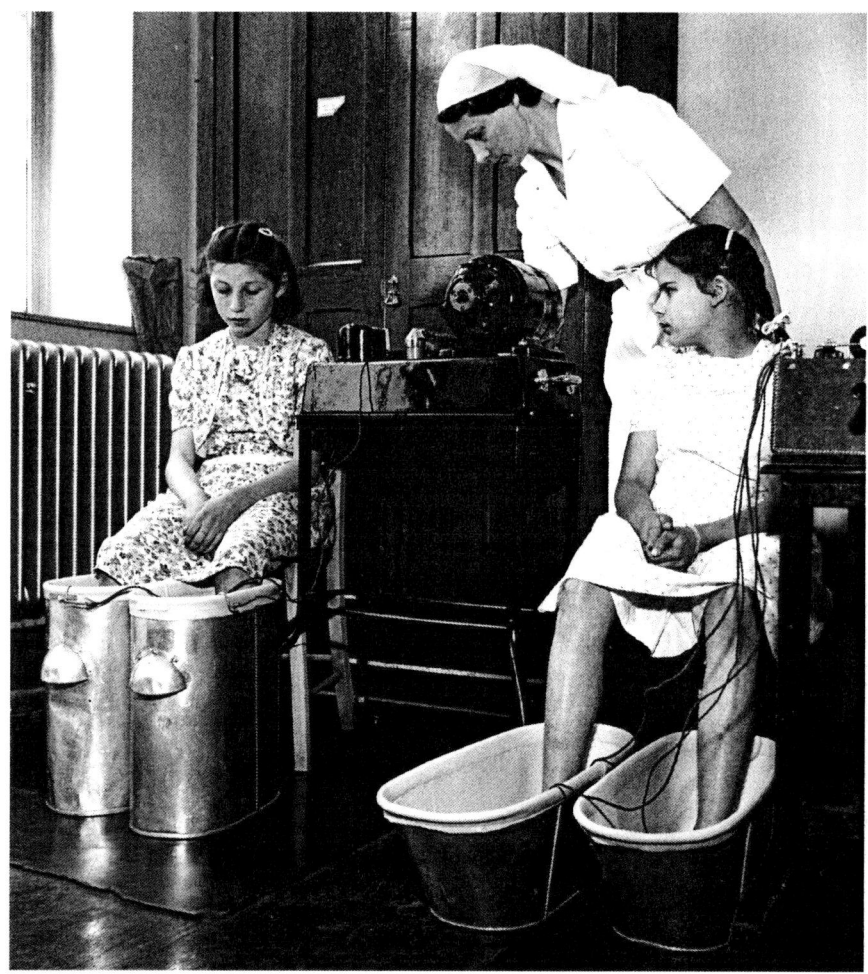

Under the newly introduced free National Health Service, a highly trained nurse at this Bristol health centre gives the girl on the right a faradic current bath for flat feet as the other young girl has a sinusoidal footbath in the centre's orthopaedic department. (Original caption).

Endnotes

(1)   C. Webster, 'The nursing crises of the early National Health Service', *Bulletin of the History of Nursing Group*, 7 (1985), p.6

(2)   T. Clay, *Nurse Power and Politics* (1987), p.70

(3)   R. White, *The Effects of the National Health Service on the Nursing Profession* (1985), p.270

(4)   R. Cooter, 'Medicine and War', in W.F. Bynum and R. Porter, eds., *The Companion Encyclopedia of the History of Medicine* (1993)

(5)   Clay, *op cit.*, p.71

(6)   RCNA. RCN/T/10. Oral history transcript, Dame Elizabeth Cockayne, March 1984

(7)   B. Abel-Smith, *A History of the Nursing Profession* (1960), p.244

(8)   White, *op cit.*

(9)   Abel-Smith, *op cit.*, p.190

(10)   R. Dingwall, A. Rafferty and C. Webster, *A Social Introduction to Nursing* (1988), p.117

(11)   RCNA. RCN/T/10. Dame E. Cockayne, oral history transcript, March 1984

(12)   *Ibid.*

(13)   R. Wood, *The Working Party into the Recruitment and Wastage of Nurses* (1947), p.iii

(14)   General Nursing Council, Memorandum concerning nurse training submitted to the Minister of Health, 1948, p.15

(15)   For a comprehensive view of this neofeudalist stance, see C. Barnett, 'The Education of Military Elites', in R. Wilkinson, ed., *Governing Elites: studies in training and selection* (New York, 1969), p.193-214

(16)   Wood, *op cit.*, p.1

(17)   *Ibid.*, p.43

(18)   *Ibid.*, p.41

(19)   *Ibid.*

(20)   *Ibid.*, p.17

(21)   *Ibid.*, p.18

(22)   Expert Committee on the Work of Psychologists and Psychiatrists in the Services (H.M.S.O. 1947)

(23)   Wood, *op cit.*, p.62

(24)   *Ibid.*, p.68

(25)   J. Cohen, *The Minority Report on the Recruitment of Nurses* (1948), p.iv. For background, see A. Rafferty, *The Politics of Nursing Knowledge* (1996)

(26)   Cohen, *op cit.*, p.v

(27)   *Ibid.*, p.73-4

(28)   *Ibid.*, p.64

(29)   *Ibid.*, p.69

(30)   *Ibid.*, p.70

(31)   *Ibid.*

(32)   *Ibid.*

(33)   *Ibid.*, p.71

(34)   *Ibid.*, p.66

(35)   *Ibid.*, p.65

(36)   *Ibid.*, p.65

(37)   *British Nursing Journal*, editorial, November 1948

(38)   RCN/T/10. Dame Elizabeth Cockayne, oral history transcript, 1984

(39)   *Parliamentary Debates* (House of Lords), 5th ser., 158, 23rd September 1948 col.228

(40)   White, *op cit.*, p.49

(41)   *Parliamentary Debates* (House of Commons), 5th ser., 469, 4th November 1949, col.797

(42)   *Parliamentary Debates* (House of Commons), 5th ser., 468, 28th October 1949, col.1667

(43)   White, *op cit.*, p.49

(44)   Dingwall *et al*, *op cit.*, p.120

(45)   White, *op cit.*, p.50. White's assumption does not appear to have any foundation whatsoever.

(46)   RCN/13/ED/1. Dame Kathleen Raven, oral history transcript, March 1988.

(47)   Dingwall *et al*, *op cit.*, p.120

(48)   Dame Kathleen Raven, *op cit.*

(49)   Dame Elizabeth Cockayne, *op cit.*

(50)   Abel-Smith, *op cit.*, p.216

(51)   Dame Elizabeth Cockayne, *op cit.*

(52)   *British Nursing Journal*, April 1948, p.48

(53)   *Ibid.*

(54)   PRO MH/55/2074. Letter to the Minister of Health from the Secretary of the Socialist Medical Association.

(55)   Great Ormond Street Nursing Advisory Minutes, 16th September 1947

(56)   Dame Elizabeth Cockayne, *op cit.*

(57)   White, *op cit.*, p.29

(58)   *Ibid.*, p.15

(59)   Clay, *op cit.*, p.72

(60)   A new syllabus was introduced to capitalise on the reintroduction of a minimum educational level for nurse training in 1962. More theory was included in the syllabus, with an emphasis on crossover education between the mental and general nursing fields.

(61)   Abel-Smith, *op cit.*, p.266

(62)   Cohen, *op cit.*, p.iv

(63)   A. Briggs, *Report of the Committee on Nursing* (1972), p.31

Chapter 4

Changing the Pattern

Nursing shortages were estimated to be in the range of 40,000 to 50,000[1] during the early stages of National Health Service development and government officials were, not surprisingly, more concerned with nurse recruitment than with nurse reform; although it could be argued that the latter may have improved the former. Unfortunately, in the area of nurse recruitment, the obstacles to change were numerous, varied considerably within individual hospitals, and appeared to be insurmountable. The Ministry of Health, in co-operation with the Ministry of Labour, sought to effect change against a background of entrenched attitudes and nursing tradition. As a consequence, most government recruitment initiatives were blocked at hospital level. Even so, the reports of both Wood and Cohen, rejected by the nursing establishment, were nonetheless extremely influential in dictating government recruitment policy in the post-war period. Wood had argued that nursing recruitment levels could be significantly improved by encouraging men to enter the profession and by the introduction of part-time nurses. Therefore, prompted by Wood's analysis, the Ministry of Labour attempted to change the nature and pattern of the nursing workforce accordingly. Cohen, meanwhile, had highlighted the need for further research and numerous surveys were conducted to determine the most effective recruitment method. Moreover, since both reports had stressed the connection between nurse discipline and high student wastage rates, the Ministry of Health concentrated on improving staff relationships. These strategies, however, represented long-term solutions to the nurse recruitment problems; government officials preparing for the emergence of the NHS were confronted by an acute shortage of labour. This situation was compounded by the lack of accurate statistical information regarding hospitals, doctors and nurses. Arbitrary figures were supplied by local authorities and health departments in an attempt to estimate future nursing requirements, but these were not reliable. Mr Isaacs at the Ministry of Labour stated in 1947 that 'October last my department had particulars of over 32,000 vacancies for nurses and over 6,500 vacancies for domestics, most of which were in hospitals'.[2] However, despite this statement and the information contained in the Majority and Minority reports, it was impossible to predict with any degree of accuracy how many nurses would be needed to staff the health service. As Dr Cohen asserted in 1948:

We are rather in the position of an architect 'planning a house' without knowing either the size of the edifice, the materials and labour required or the number and variety of people who are to live in it. [3]

Furthermore, this position failed to be clarified with time:

In 1969 the Committee of Public Accounts was concerned that health departments did not know whether there were too many or too few nurses - 20 years after the NHS came into being. [4]

Nevertheless, while officials deliberated over future nursing requirements of the health service, the immediate nursing shortage was obvious. On 7th September 1945 four nursing sisters from the West Middlesex Hospital travelled to Whitehall and demanded an audience with the Minister of Health. The sisters presented a letter to Bevan's secretary and were duly given an appointment to be received by the Minister of Health on Monday 11th September. The letter which the sisters left on behalf of the trained staff of their own hospital and hospitals in general made the following five points:

1. We are unable to continue any longer under the present conditions of acute staff shortage. The nature of our profession makes it impossible for us to strike. As a result we are being exploited.

2. Patients are being inadequately nursed. Wards are constantly left in the care of inexperienced and junior nurses.

3. Trained nurses stay on voluntarily long after scheduled hours. Owing to the scarcity of domestics, nurses have to clean wards and wash up.

4. The staffing problem could be alleviated by the early release of trained nurses from the Forces and a new method of allocating nurses when training is completed.

5. There is insufficient difference in pay between a student nurse in her last year and the staff nurse and ward sister. There is too great a difference in pay between the ward sister and the matron [5]

Recruitment Problems: The Initial Solution

During the meeting with the West Middlesex nursing sisters, Bevan revealed that he was fully aware of the difficulties confronting the nursing profession:

He was in consultation with the Minister of Labour and National Service as to the possibility of securing an acceleration in the release of nurses from the Armed Forces. Efforts were also being made to encourage male nursing orderlies, on demobilisation from the RAMC, to enter hospital service, and the Ministry of Labour and National Service had launched a new recruitment campaign for hospital staff, in which a special appeal would be made to women leaving the Services and war industry. [6]

Consequently, by 31st March 1946 39,000 nursing orderlies and VADs were released from military service, and a further 41,000 were awaiting release at a later date.[7] In addition, between June 1945 and December 1947, 19,651 female nursing members were released from the Armed Forces nursing services.[8]

All military personnel were offered a class B demobilisation if they agreed to embark on a nursing career and special rates of pay were introduced. Bevan also launched an appeal to persuade nurses released in the class A category from the forces to return immediately to civilian nursing. Intensive one-year registration courses were reluctantly established by the GNC 'to encourage more men and women who have had substantial nursing experience in the Services to make civilian nursing their career'.[9] The GNC had argued that ex-service nursing orderlies would find intensive registration courses too difficult; in fact, examination results did not bear out these assumptions since the number of passes - 91.1% - exceeded the normal pass rate for nurse training. In addition to intensive courses and quicker demobilisation for military personnel choosing to enter the civilian nursing profession, a reduction of six months in the registration training period was awarded to ex-service orderlies and VADs who were not eligible to undertake intensive courses.

These concessions by the GNC to ex-service personnel were not withdrawn until 1953 and the influx of nursing recruits from demobilised forces greatly alleviated staff shortages. In 1945, nursing shortages resulted in the closure of 30,000 hospital beds but, as Dame Elizabeth recalled, 'There was no shortage after the war because of all those returning from military service'.[10] However, while large numbers of ex-service personnel did take advantage of government incentives, it is impossible to assess the number of people who signed contracts for registration training merely to obtain early release from military service and perhaps abandoned training at the earliest opportunity. There were also difficulties associated with the intensive one-year registration courses; hospitals were not given additional funds by the Ministry of Health to run these courses and a severe shortage of sister tutors prevented many hospitals, particularly those in rural areas, from taking full advantage of demobilised personnel. The first intensive courses were established in 'Nottingham, Manchester, Newcastle, Leeds, Birmingham, London and Bristol between 1946 and 1947'.[11]

Intensive training courses were based on the primacy of general nursing. Demobilised personnel hoping to become registered mental nurses by means of such courses were disappointed. The Ministry of Health had initially organised reduced training schemes for the care of the mentally ill but, according to government officials, these schemes were abandoned because of administrative difficulties. The War Office had already trained 1,200 male mental nurses, and by the end of 1946 had released 520 of these. It was argued, therefore, that the number of vacancies for trained mental nurses did not justify the need for intensive courses in this area. This argument was not based on fact; as Wood had pointed out, 'the shortage of nurses is perhaps more acute in the mental field than in any other'.[12] Dame Elizabeth also observed that, in comparison with mental hospitals, 'the situation in general hospitals was relatively so much better'.[13]

Faced with such an obvious demand for trained mental nurses, the failure to introduce intensive training programmes in this field was indefensible. Administrative problems, which had been cited as the main reason for this failure, centred on the fact that, prior to 1948, mental healthcare was administered by the Home Office. The duality of the training system also gave rise to some confusion. A person was able to qualify as a mental nurse either by passing GNC examinations or those of the Royal Medico-Psychological Association (RMPA). For various reasons, both of these groups were reluctant to administer one-year courses in mental nursing. The RMPA planned to relinquish its role as an examining board for mental nurses and did so in 1951. The GNC exhibited an overwhelming bias towards the training of general nurses and argued that a shortage of suitable tutors precluded any action in the area of mental health. Consequently, ex-service personnel experienced in the care of the mentally ill were denied the opportunity to obtain registration by means of intensive training.

However, there were also nursing members of demobilised forces who, through no fault of their own, were not eligible for one-year general registration courses. According to GNC guidelines, applicants for intensive training 'must have had not less than two years' experience in the nursing of the physically sick in a hospital under the supervision of registered nurses or trained nurses'.[14] In theory, eligible personnel had received training to RAMC standard ATC 344 and comprised of: (a) leading sick berth attendants; (b) class 1 nursing orderlies; and (c) leading aircraftsmen and women working as nursing orderlies. Unfortunately, the two-year hospital experience rule effectively excluded all personnel who had been engaged primarily in field service. As War Office representatives argued in 1951, 'the exigencies of the service (the outbreak of the Korean War was cited) prevented many men from obtaining the certificate ATC 344 although they might have received equivalent training'.[15] Moreover, it could be argued that experience gained in the field was far more valuable than that which could be gained in an ordinary hospital ward.

As a prerequisite for course eligibility, trained nurse supervision was also an unfair GNC demand since civilian student nurses frequently worked unsupervised. Furthermore, compared to many civilian hospitals, the Services provided a higher standard of nurse training. Mr McAlpine, on behalf of the Ministry of Labour and National Service, stressed that government policy regarding ex-service personnel insisted that training gained in the forces should not be discounted by civilian employers. Nevertheless, despite these valid arguments, eligibility rules for courses were not relaxed and the GNC remained intransigent.

In May 1947 there were 537 ex-military personnel attending one-year registration courses - 173 females and 364 males. Sixteen training centres had been established and the demand for courses continued until 1951, when applicants began to diminish in number. Ex-military nursing staff considered ineligible for one-year courses opted for nurse training schemes offering a six-month concession, and many orderlies with field experience joined the ambulance service.

The influx of demobilised personnel into the nursing services, however, did not consist entirely of new recruits. Many senior nurses were required to enter military service during the war and, once demobilised, frequently returned to the same senior positions. Hospitals managed to retain nurses by agreeing to meet superannuation payments for the duration of their military service, providing they returned to the hospital concerned on demobilisation, and had taken the view that 'those members who were called up for service with the Forces would be reinstated at the conclusion of hostilities if they so desired'.[16]

While hospitals made concerted efforts to retain their trained nursing staff, matrons also endeavoured to recruit ex-service orderlies to work as auxiliaries. The reasoning behind this recruitment drive was clear; the demand for untrained nursing staff had increased rapidly due to the shortage of trained nurses. Since there was no recognised civilian training course for auxiliaries, the only way to obtain auxiliaries with nursing experience and training was by recruiting ex-service personnel.

Despite this rapid increase in untrained nursing staff, professional nursing organisations and the Ministry of Health did not consider it necessary to introduce some elementary training, although the Ministry did concede that some training might be useful in the mental sector. As Abel-Smith noted:

> *Short courses of training had been laid down for auxiliaries working in the war time Voluntary Aid Detachments; even in peacetime first-aid training was given to those whose services would be needed in a possible war and in the army itself basic nursing continued to be taught in brief courses to nursing orderlies. Schemes of training in the National Health Service extended from the administrators to the stokers; there were no formal courses for nursing auxiliaries.* [17]

This situation continued and, although some hospitals introduced training courses, they were very rudimentary. A nurse working in Manchester recalled that 'we gave the auxiliaries a week's good training to take temperatures and handle patients'.[18] The lack of training for auxiliaries had severe implications for student nurses. Since trained supervision was not always available, it was the auxiliaries and not the ward sisters who explained nursing procedures to new students, a problem which may have contributed to student wastage rates but one which did not appear to concern the government nor professional organisations:

> *The NHS, like the First World War generals, came to rely on a steady stream of eager, cheap, obedient recruits who formed the backbone of the workforce and were replaced in due course by another cohort.* [19]

Although demobilised forces had alleviated the immediate nursing crisis in the NHS, long-term action was needed to prevent further nursing shortages. The government, therefore, in addition to traditional recruitment methods, implemented the recruitment strategies outlined by Wood. As previously acknowledged, these strategies were aimed at wooing married women back to the profession by the introduction of part-time shifts and by encouraging the employment of male nurses. Reducing nurse wastage rates was also a primary objective and ministers fully appreciated that these rates were linked to poor staff relationships. In an effort to combat this problem, notes for hospital guidance in employing nurses were circulated, drawing attention to the fact that:

The staffing of hospitals can be seriously prejudiced by bad staff relations, e.g. inadequate training methods, the 'institutional' attitude of senior staff, repressive discipline, out-moded social distinctions between grades of staff (especially between trained and student nurses and part-time and full-time staff) and restrictions on the personal freedom of nurses when off duty. [20]

Nevertheless, while government officials were aware of the problems, policies designed to both improve recruitment levels and reduce wastage rates met with varying degrees of success and relied heavily on the co-operation of individual hospitals. Furthermore, the nursing profession itself exhibited considerable hostility towards part-time nurses and appeared reluctant to employ men in the general nursing sphere. Matrons tended to prefer a young, female, compliant workforce and to this end frequently relied on child labour and an immigrant workforce to staff the hospitals. However, in order to fully determine the success of government recruitment policy, it is necessary to examine certain strategies in more depth. Therefore, the following analysis will focus on male nursing, part-time nursing, immigrant nursing and child labour.

Recruitment Problems: Long-term Solutions

Bringing in the men

According to official statistics, by 1949 one-in-five nurses were male whereas, before the war, the figure had been one-in-ten.[21] However, Ministry of Health statistics were not reliable and these figures did not distinguish between mental and general nurses or between trained and untrained staff. The figures for the number of general nurses registered by examination with the GNC in 1945 claim that a total of 7,157 females qualified compared to a total of 29 men.[22] Even taking into account the introduction of intensive courses in general nursing from 1946 onwards, the Ministry of Health figures were not correct when applied to the general nursing sphere. Brown and Stone estimated that by 1950 'there were 25,600 male nurses trained and untrained constituting 17 per cent of the total nursing labour force'.[23] The majority of male nurses were still to be found in the mental health field and many believed they should remain there.

This resistance to the concept of male general nurses was not confined to professional spheres. While, in theory, government ministers accepted the need for male nurses, many expressed serious doubts as to whether the general public would welcome such a fundamental change. As Lord Crook announced in the House of Lords:

> *I stand here in the very difficult role of advocating the employment of male nurses while being quite certain that I like having had my brow smoothed by a ministering angel of the female sex. So we share that view of nursing. I regret that the economic situation and the manpower situation of the country force me to suggest such outrageous things as taking away ministering angels and substituting male nurses.* [24]

This sentiment was echoed throughout parliamentary debates and expressed succinctly in the following statement:

> *Men nurses for mental cases and for other specialised forms of attention of course are quite right; but I do not know about general nursing. Perhaps it is only the sentimental attitude of a man who, fortunately, in his own case is hardly ever ill, but I am inclined to think that I would get better more quickly if I too had a ministering angel of the female sex. I question whether even the best trained man would do quite as well for me.* [25]

Traditional prejudices and gender expectations were difficult to overcome and while the 1949 Nurses Act had allowed for the amalgamation of the male register with that of the general register, this did not mean the end of discrimination against male nurses. The RCN did not include men until 1960 and the major London teaching hospitals did not accept men for general nurse training until 1966.[26] The British Nursing Journal expressed the views of some female nurses in a lengthy editorial:

> *For many years now women have struggled to gain equality with men in the world of employment. In all the long bitter struggle there has been one sphere where the right of employment was never questioned - the nursing profession. Inevitably, it seems, with the reshuffling of the sexes in the employment world, men have come knocking at the doors of the nursing profession. We can look on with sympathy, albeit with some amusement, to see the reversal of the struggle we have so long participated in.* [27]

The editorial continued by describing all the problems associated with male nurses. For instance, men were only allowed to administer care to male patients, a policy that restricted their employment opportunities. Consequently, many male nurses gravitated towards the tutorial field, a move which challenged the female power base in this area. However, according to the nursing press, female nurses could afford to be magnanimous. Men:

> ... will have to realise that to compete with women in their own sphere other than at a time of shortage of candidates, will not be easy for them. Men will have to realise more than they seem to do now, that there is more in ward management than the treatment of the patients, before they will be a serious threat to women's supremacy as ward sisters. If men could bring into their wards the order and cleanliness of a crack ship as well as their noted thoroughness, any matron would have a ward charge nurse to delight her.[28]

In view of the public and professional prejudice that surrounded the issue of male nursing, men, not surprisingly, needed to be firmly convinced that general nursing offered them a worthwhile career. Mental nursing had required physical strength in order to restrain patients; it was therefore an acceptable male profession. General nursing was associated with soothing gentle care and most definitely considered to be a feminine profession, added to which, even if a man managed to overcome the obstacles of prejudice and rise to the top of the general nursing hierarchy, there were few men who aspired to the title of 'male matron'. However, senior nurses at the Ministry of Health and the Ministry of Labour tackled the prejudice problem on two fronts: firstly, various incentives were introduced to entice men into general nursing; and secondly, hospitals were made aware that employing male nurses did have certain advantages.

By 1950 the Nursing Appointments Service of the Ministry of Labour had expanded and included 135 officers. In addition, technical nursing officers were available to encourage suitable applicants to enter the profession. Recruitment posters targeting men were displayed at employment exchanges, along with leaflets explaining the generous nurse training allowances available for men and their dependants. It was also possible for men to defer their call-up for National Service by entering the nursing profession. However, hospitals argued that generally 'male applicants were of rather poor quality, though ex-service personnel were good'.[29] There was also a problem with accommodation. It was not always possible for hospitals to provide the married or family accommodation frequently demanded by male applicants.

However, as nurses at the Ministry of Health maintained, although accommodation presented difficulties it was worth overcoming these in order to gain male staff. As the notes for guidance of the Hospital Management Committee explained:

HMCs should consider whether they might not profitably increase the number of male nurses employed, bearing in mind the longer average period of service obtainable from men than from women. [30]

It was this fact that provided the most convincing argument in favour of employing male general nurses. Since male nurses were more likely than females to have dependants, it was argued that they would, from necessity, be more committed to nursing as a career, whereas many women left the profession on marriage, never to return.

The government recruitment strategies appeared to be very successful, but the willingness to employ male nurses was often dictated by the availability of alternative labour. Standard hospital recruitment practice ensured that in most cases female nurses took precedence over male nurses. There were occasions, however, when male nurses were specifically requested by hospitals. Consultant surgeons at the Royal London Hospital had not approved of female nurses running the theatre during the war. Rather than continue with the arrangement, surgeons insisted that male nurses should be appointed. Two male nurses were duly appointed, but one 'had found the work in the theatres too much for him and he had resigned after a period of six months to take a post in a smaller hospital'.[31]

By the 1950s many hospitals were in the process of overcoming prejudiced attitudes towards men. The General Purposes Committee of the United Oxford Hospitals Group, for instance, announced that it had 'no objection to the employment of male nurses in general hospitals in any grade, including that of charge nurse'.[32] However, there were indications that the numbers of male nurse recruits were dwindling at the very point when prejudice against them was subsiding. This was partly due to the fact that shortened courses for ex-service personnel were disbanded in 1953 and partly because men were now competing with an ever-increasing immigrant population. In 1954:

The number of female student nurses in training increased by 196 but the number of males fell by 314 and there was therefore a net reduction in the total number of student nurses from 48,292 to 48,174. There was only a slight increase in the numbers of whole time trained male nurses from 12,038 to 12,052. The numbers of whole time trained female nurses on the other hand increased substantially from 37,588 to 38,382. [33]

Until the abolition of National Service, ex-service personnel continued to provide the main source of male nurse recruits. Indeed, many hospitals had established strong links with ex-servicemen's associations specifically to aid the recruitment process. The most important development to affect the influx of male nurses, however, centred on the restructuring of senior nursing grades in the late 1960s. The restructuring of administrative posts advocated by the Salmon report opened up a variety of clinical grades and promotional prospects. Salmon also gave senior nurses new 'officer' titles; the 'male matron' therefore became obsolete and was replaced by the 'chief nursing officer'. Within two years of the implementation of the Salmon recommendations, men occupied one-third of all senior posts![34] Contrary to the earlier predictions made by the *British Nursing Journal*, men did in fact successfully challenge women's supremacy on the wards.

Continuity of care: the issue of part-time nursing

In view of the severe labour shortage in the post-war years, government policy towards women was aimed at encouraging as many as possible into the workplace, and the practice of employing part-time nurses had already gained a degree of acceptance during the war years. However, matrons had considered this practice a matter of wartime expediency. They argued that, in the interests of continuity of patient care, part-time nursing should not become acceptable in peacetime. This argument was not particularly valid; many hospitals had been forced to employ agency nurses to cope with staff shortages. These nurses were shifted from ward to ward and, consequently, rarely administered care to the same patients. Employing permanent nurses on a part-time basis, therefore, allocated to one specific ward, would have provided more continuity in care than that supplied by agency nurses. Nevertheless, matrons were not convinced, they believed that married women had divided interests and would be unable to concentrate on their work. Nursing required total dedication and a sense of duty; part-time nurses, it was argued, particularly those with children, could not possibly provide this commitment. With regard to pregnant nurses, most matrons continued to assume that nurses 'had no intention of returning once the baby was born'.[35] Some hospitals experimented with part-time nurses but claimed they usually abandoned work after a period of six months because they found it difficult to cope with work and family responsibilities.

Nurses at Whitehall recognised that hospitals needed to alleviate some of the domestic problems encountered by married women and advised ministers accordingly. Consequently, Ministry of Health guidelines for the employment of married women in hospitals advised that:

> *... the welfare of part-time workers should be given consideration, women who would normally cook for themselves and families will appreciate a well cooked meal when on duty. Meals on duty should be provided free of charge and working uniform should be provided and laundered free of charge.* [36]

Government officials insisted that hospitals should make every effort to attract married women back to work and, since Ministry of Labour recruitment posters boldly claimed that 'if you have nursing training or experience, you can return to your hospital work without serious disruption of your private life as a wife, mother or homeworker',[37] hospitals were at the very least required to pay lip service to the welfare concerns of part-time women.

The poster campaigns were very successful in attracting potential recruits and numerous women appeared eager to maintain their nursing career through part-time work. However, despite concerted efforts by the Ministry of Labour, these women were frequently denied a hospital post simply because matrons did not approve of part-time nursing. Acknowledging this resistance, a Ministry official stated, 'The fault I fear lies with the matrons who obviously were, and are still quite lukewarm about part-time nursing'.[38] An analysis of the Royal London Hospital staffing figures (shown in Table 4.1) reveals that part-time nurses were not widely employed, even by the mid 1950s. It was also clear from studying the nursing advisory minutes in several hospitals that part-time staff were only considered for posts if they had completed their training at the employing hospital. This elitist and restrictive employment practice continued well into the 1960s. Moreover, part-time nurses were usually employed in areas such as outpatients or radiography clinics to avoid changing shift times.

Since matrons were lukewarm towards employing part-time nurses, it was not surprising that when the Ministry of Labour suggested the possibility of part-time training in 1955, the reaction was positively hostile. A review conducted by the Ministry of Labour's National Advisory Council for the Recruitment of Nurses and Midwives suggested that part-time training would act as a great stimulus to recruitment from the ranks of auxiliaries and from women who had not previously undertaken nursing work. Many good candidates were lost to the nursing profession, they argued, simply because they

Table 4.1 Total nursing staff, selected dates, 1953-6

27 July 1953	Full-Time	Part-Time
Sisters	133	0
Staff nurses	131	0
Student nurses	505	0
Total nursing staff	**769**	**0**

26 July 1954	Full-Time	Part-Time
Sisters	134	3
Staff nurses (including midwives)	130	9
Pupil midwives	18	0
Student nurses	516	0
Others (assistant and pre-training)	17	1
Total nursing staff	**815**	**13**

28 November 1955	Full-Time	Part-Time
Sisters	123	4
Staff midwives	13	1
Staff nurses	78	14
Pupil midwives	32	0
Student nurses	543	0
Others (assistant and pre-training)	3	2
Total nursing staff	**792**	**21**

23 April 1956	Full-Time	Part-Time
Sisters	127	3
Staff midwives	17	1
Staff nurses	92	13
Pupil midwives	39	0
Student nurses	549	0
Assistants	4	3
Pre-training	20	0
Total nursing staff	**848**	**20**

Source: Royal London Hospital nursing minutes.

were unable to train full-time. The Council had also observed that students frequently abandoned training in their third year to get married; if these students could continue their training on a part-time basis they would not be lost to the profession. Predictably:

> ... the opinions expressed by the professional bodies concerned made it clear, however, that they would have difficulty in accepting the principle of part-time training, chiefly because they considered the candidate would, by reason of her divided interests and home ties, be unable to give proper attention to her training and would not be ready to do her share of the less popular chores.

Nevertheless, despite nursing protestations, objections to part-time nurses did not actually centre on the 'divided interest' argument, nor on the 'continuity of care' argument. The primary objection revolved around organisational problems. Ward sisters were not inclined to rearrange shifts and, as a nursing officer working with the Manchester Regional Health Board explained, if part-time nurses claim. [39]

... we can only work from six until eight or two until five whatever, if you need nurses in your hospital (this was my theory never put into practice) you must put yourself out to fit in with their demands, they're going to be a useful pair of hands; even if it means reorganising things a bit on the wards. [40]

This view was echoed by the Ministry of Health, which argued that 'the secret of the successful use of part-time staff lies in organising work to suit the individual circumstances of the workers'.[41]

'Between 1946 and May 1955 the number of married women in gainful employment rose by two and a quarter million to three and three quarter million',[42] and by the mid 1960s hospitals were becoming more amenable to the idea of employing nurses on a flexible basis. However, while government policy generally was aimed at encouraging married women back to work in all areas of employment, local authorities in many areas had reduced their nursery provision.[43] Commenting on this problem in the House of Commons, Mr Pardoe, a Liberal MP, stated that:

The employment in industry of women, particularly housewives and mothers of young children, presents a problem. Not only do we want to bring back those qualified as doctors and teachers - the need is obvious - but we want to bring women into employment in the whole length and breadth of British industry. We all know about the 'latch key' children and we don't want to encourage that sort of thing. We should ensure that industry is able to adapt itself to the problems of housewives and mothers of young children. [44]

Ministers continued to discuss the childcare problems of working mothers, but no real action was taken to resolve them. Similarly, ministers debated the taxation system but decided that changes to the system would have little impact on working women.

To some extent, the views of married nurses supported government opinion. A survey of trained married nurses conducted in 1967 revealed that 'flexibility of hours and better childcare facilities were more important than improved pay for women wanting to return'.[45] However, although the field of general nursing consisted of a predominantly female workforce, surprisingly the profession made no allowances for the fact that many nurses would have dependants and failed to respond to the fundamental need for childcare. As Clay observed, nursing exhibited 'its own brand of discrimination against women'[46] and it was arguably this discrimination which allowed men to gain access to professional power. While the nursing profession was 'numerically dominated by women, the road to advancement is through a model in which the man committed to full-time work is given a head start'.[47] Consequently, power positions within the profession were restricted to those women able to provide continuous service. Nursing had failed to provide the support networks necessary to achieve flexibility in care provision and promotional opportunities for women with domestic responsibilities. Despite government efforts to the contrary, matrons and sisters had rejected the part-time labour force throughout the 1950s and 1960s and concentrated instead on recruiting full-time immigrant labour.

Pure European descent: recruiting overseas nurses

Thus far, analysis of nurse recruitment has emphasised government attempts to change the nature of the nursing workforce in the face of considerable resistance. The issue of recruiting immigrant labour, however, presents a totally different picture in that matrons actively encouraged the recruitment of immigrant labour. Nursing shortages were first alleviated by the recruitment of overseas workers during the war and they were commonly referred to as 'aliens'. By the late 1940s, sixteen British colonies had established selection and recruitment procedures to ensure a steady intake of colonial nurse recruits for the NHS. In addition:

> Enterprising matrons set off for the Caribbean, West Africa and the Philippines to recruit labour. In some cases they were so successful that you could find hospitals where almost all the staff below the rank of sister were of ethnic minority. [48]

These matrons were motivated primarily by a desperate need to staff their hospitals, but there were other considerations. Hospital accommodation for nurses was of a relatively poor standard in the post-war years and nurses were still required to work long hours. There appeared to be a general assumption that immigrants recruited to the nursing services were less likely to complain about accommodation problems and working conditions than their British counterparts. This view had emerged with the British refugee policy during the war. However, 'philanthropy in helping to rescue the Jewish women was not incompatible with exploitation'.[49] Similarly, immigrant labour incorporated into the nursing profession was also subject to exploitation.

The way in which immigrant labour was perceived in post-war Britain largely reflected the legacy of the Empire and the nursing profession codified racial prejudice along the lines of long-standing military policy. For years the British military had insisted that all recruits were of 'pure British descent'. This later became 'pure European descent' and, although the RAF was forced to temporarily rescind this policy due to a shortage of pilots during the war, racism was nevertheless an inherent feature of the British military and one which became codified within civilian society. Consequently, public reaction to black labour differed fundamentally from responses to European labour, therefore:

> ... the degree of toleration eventually addressed to European volunteer workers in the immediate post-war period should not be seen as indicating a similar response towards New Commonwealth migrants, settling in Britain at the same time. [50]

The Minister of Labour, George Isaacs, was fully aware of the codification process and the fact that public attitudes encapsulated 'a particular set of values about a hierarchy of 'races', one which was to be made abundantly clear in post-war Britain'.[51]

It was also abundantly clear that, while nursing ethics supposedly endorsed a policy of administering care to patients equally, irrespective of class, colour or creed,[52] nurses did not extend this policy of equality to members of their own profession. As early as 1948 the Minister of Health:

> ... dissociated himself from the action of a London matron who had imposed a colour bar at a dance in respect of one of her own nursing staff, a colonial citizen working in the best interest of the London community. [53]

This action by a London matron was not an isolated incident and, while hospitals needed immigrant labour, they did not necessarily respect immigrants as equal members of the workforce. Moreover, the hierarchy of 'races' was visible in the recruitment practices of most hospitals, with 'black' and Irish nurses appearing at the bottom of the hierarchical order. Although there was some evidence to suggest that Irish recruits did not suffer the same exploitation as blacks, instead they frequently voted with their feet and abandoned the profession. Since the travel expenses of these Irish nurses had been met by the Ministry of Labour, the policy of recruiting women from Ireland was severely criticised by Members of Parliament, although registers suggest that Irish nurses did remain in the English labour market after leaving the profession. Immigration policy, however, continually exposed a variety of inconsistencies between government departments. For instance, relatives of Jewish refugees were refused entry to Britain in the post-war years in accordance with the Distressed Relatives Scheme administered by the Home Office, while the Ministry of Labour had:

> ... recognised that the Home Office scheme to help those Jews who had survived the war on the continent was highly restrictive. It thus turned a blind eye to applicants turned down by the Home Office who now wanted to come under the Ministry's foreign domestic worker scheme. [54]

Since the shortage of domestic labour affected the work and recruitment of nurses, obtaining immigrants to work in this area remained a priority throughout the post-war era.

Analysis of hospital nurses' registers reveals that a large majority of nurses working in British hospitals in the 1950s and 1960s came from overseas, and countries of origin included India, Germany, Belgium, France, Greece, Holland, Switzerland, Jamaica and South Africa. Furthermore, 'the most rapid increase in the number of immigrant nurses and midwives was between 1959 and 1964'.[55] In the immediate post-war period a large proportion of overseas nurses were recruited from Nigeria and the West Indies; by the 1960s, however, a shift had taken place with nurses mainly recruited from Malaysia and Mauritius. In most instances, nurses from overseas experienced severe communication problems in addition to both overt and covert forms of racial prejudice. Moreover, immigration was used by the nursing profession to reinforce existing class distinctions, thereby elevating the status of the registered nurse.

As Clay has noted, many immigrant nurse recruits were persuaded to undertake enrolled nurse training rather than training for registration. However, the second grade enrolled nurse represented:

> ... one of the health service's biggest confidence tricks. Pupil nurse courses were filled in the 1950s and 1960s by recruits from

Mauritius, the Philippines and elsewhere, who were misled into
believing they were doing a registered nurse training that would
put them on a secure career path. Too late, they discovered that
the enrolled nurse qualification was the road to nowhere in the
UK and virtually useless back home. [56]

Since immigrants, particularly those with language difficulties, were not aware of the differences in nurse training, 'channelling them into EN training was a covert form of racism'.[57] There were no promotional prospects associated with the enrolled nurse certificate and, although many immigrants possessed good educational qualifications, they were denied the opportunity to train for the register. Consequently, access to professional power could only be claimed by white, middle-class, registered nurses.

It can further be argued that immigration saved the enrolled nurse training scheme from possible extinction. As Cohen remarked in 1948, 'In spite of every effort to stimulate recruitment to this grade, the results have fallen far short of expectations and the scheme is dying a natural death'.[58] Many hospitals were reluctant to run courses for pupil nurses, as a Nursing Officer in Manchester recalled:

They thought they would lose status, the question of status came
into it, to a certain extent they just wanted to train SRNs because it
was a higher qualification, and I think they were frightened of the
type of girl who would be coming in for SEN training. [59]

Immigration secured the survival of the second grade nurse and underpinned the higher social status of the registered nurse. Since the social background of registered nurses differed substantially from that of enrolled nurses throughout this period, there may have been 'some waste of nursing ability for social reasons'.[60]

Despite the language problems associated with immigrant nurses and occasional difficulties with obtaining recruits due to fluctuations in the international labour market, matrons employed immigrant labour in preference to male and part-time nurses. The reasons for doing so were obvious - immigrant labour generally made for a compliant workforce. Dependent on their work for accommodation and livelihood, and far removed from their own culture, immigrant nurses did not initially complain about working conditions. Moreover, the widespread institutional racism in the NHS[61] ensured that immigrants were fully exploited. While government immigration policy as a whole could be interpreted as a means of maintaining a patriarchal society, within the confines of the nursing profession immigration was a means of maintaining class distinctions.

Recruiting the children?
The policy of recruiting nurses from overseas had in many respects obscured the fact that the numbers of native-born 18-year-old girls was falling and that fewer of these girls were choosing nursing as a career. Moreover, the practice of diverting overseas nurses into enrolled rather than registration training posed significant problems with regard to nurse administration. From the mid 1950s onwards, motivated by the desire to improve efficiency in healthcare delivery, ministers were eager to reorganise the administration of nursing services. However, a continuing shortage of registered nurses undermined government plans to initiate change since it was not feasible to reorganise nurse administration without an adequate number of suitably trained nurses to fill administrative posts. In an effort to resolve this situation, the focus of government attention shifted towards the native-born nurse recruit and the issue of student wastage. It was no longer 'enough to know why ex-preliminary training school girls give up their training, but to try and find out what is in the mind of the girl before she enters the preliminary training school'.[62]

There were, however, considerable difficulties associated with assessing nurse recruitment and wastage levels, let alone trying to find out what was in young girls' minds! A complete lack of reliable data pertaining to existing recruitment levels severely hampered investigations and, even when data became available, the policy of compiling statistics as national aggregates served to obscure staffing problems which emerged on a regional basis. Furthermore, extensive research carried out by the Nuffield Trust, the Department of Industrial Administration and similar organisations had failed to devise an adequate method of determining nursing requirements. Consequently, there was 'no adequate data relating to the overall balance between nursing and midwifery supply and demand on a national level'.[63] Attempts to clarify the position revealed a mass of statistical anomalies. For instance, there were several discrepancies between the figures supplied by the Ministry of Labour and those supplied by the Ministry of Health as the means of calculating statistics differed between departments. The Ministry of Health based recruitment needs on 'the return calls for the number of vacancies at a given date, whereas the Ministry of Labour figure was based on the number required for the next preliminary training school'[64] and cadet nurses were not even included in the nursing statistics.

It was this séction of the nursing workforce, excluded from statistical analysis, which became the centre of attention in terms of 'finding out what was in a young girl's mind' before she entered the nursing profession. As Chambers noted in 1960:

> *The impact of hospital cadet schemes on the recruitment and wastage of nurses cannot be overestimated. They are a most valuable source of recruitment for student nurses and the hospital experience and educational background which the course provides fits them for a nursing career thereby reducing the wastage of student nurses from the nurses' training school.* [65]

As previously acknowledged in Chapter 2, cadet schemes inspired by military recruitment practice had emerged during the war and were designed to bridge the age gap between leaving school and entering nurse training. However, the quality of cadet schemes varied considerably between individual hospitals and, as Baly recalled, 'most schemes in reality were merely exploiting children'.[66]

There was also a certain amount of ambiguity surrounding the role of cadets within the hospital framework. On one level, cadet work was mundane and unskilled (they delivered messages between departments and helped with cleaning, sewing, cooking and filing) while on another level, they were expected to suture wounds and attend post mortems:

> *One cadet of under sixteen years of age was feeding premature babies with a tube after they came out of the incubators. All the other girls were giving out bedpans and cleaning them and collecting and sorting dirty laundry. One girl helped to lift patients back to bed from theatre and stayed with patients until they came round from the anaesthetic.* [67]

The Ministry of Health had introduced guidelines for the employment of hospital cadets, but these were difficult to enforce. For instance, despite the fact that guidelines suggested that cadets should only work between the hours of 8.00am and 6.00pm if they were under the age of sixteen, hospitals frequently employed cadets on night duty to alleviate staffing shortages. A similar situation arose in relation to work allocation. While cadets were only permitted to undertake the duties 'clearly laid down by the Ministry of Health and by the Regional Hospital Board, in many hospitals cadets are doing tasks they are not supposed to do'.[68] Nevertheless, although cadets were undoubtedly exploited, research studies concluded that wastage rates were considerably lower amongst student nurses with cadet experience than those without. However, this research was fundamentally flawed, partly because it was concentrated in one region (northwest England) but, more importantly, in that only hospitals which had consented to participation in studies were examined. Since the level of child exploitation was likely to be more serious within the hospitals that refused to participate in research, these conclusions regarding wastage rates were meaningless. Neither did studies shed much light on the 'mind of young girls' entering the nursing profession. Cadets had complained of 'boredom, a sense of frustration with the quality of teaching and the fact that they were constantly reminded of their inferior status.[69] However, many girls had joined cadet schemes simply because they had relatives already working in the nursing profession and not necessarily from a strong desire to nurse. Those who later abandoned the schemes did so for virtually the same reasons as student nurses who abandoned training. The majority of recruits left nursing primarily because they could not cope with intolerable levels of discipline and the restrictions imposed on their private lives.

According to the representatives of various teaching organisations, it was precisely these problems, responsible for high wastage, which also prevented girls from choosing nursing as a career. The Headmasters Association had acknowledged:

> ... *terrifying stories of untrained nurses being left in charge of wards at night and to long hours, poor pay and the old-fashioned attitudes of some matrons who rule with a rod of iron. Likewise, the National Association of Head Teachers stated bluntly that neither high ideals nor long-term rewards will attract new recruits to the profession or retain them if they do wish to enter, if actual conditions are poor. The word of mouth gets around and recruitment often stands or falls by word of mouth communication between existing nurses and potential recruits.* [70]

This analysis of the nurse recruitment and wastage problems put forward by teachers was totally accurate. Nevertheless, the analysis was not new; every nursing report from 1932 onwards had cited nurse discipline and poor working conditions as a major cause of student wastage and a disincentive to recruitment. Moreover, the government had tried to improve the situation by making strong appeals to matrons and hospitals to relax 'off duty' restrictions on nurses and discard outmoded notions of discipline. Ministry appeals, however, were usually ignored along with the Ministry guidelines.

While government policy was directed at changing recruitment patterns and improving staff relationships, recruitment campaigns launched by the nursing profession continued to focus on military traditions. Campaigns during the 1950s were designed to coincide with 'civil defence weeks', stressing the heroic nature of nursing. Moreover, a popular recruitment film made by the Royal London Hospital in 1968 was shown to school children nationally, entitled *Not so much a training, more a way of life* - the film began with the arrest of Edith Cavell in 1915! The film also emphasised that nurses' uniforms at the Royal London were designed by Hartnell and that nursing as an occupation provided a practical training that was useful grounding for running a home and family. Furthermore, since potential nurse recruits continued to be more attracted to military rather than civilian nursing circles, recruitment propaganda emphasised the travel opportunities which supposedly existed for civilian nurses, for example on cruise ships and within organised holiday camps. Amid these attempts to woo intelligent young recruits, the nursing profession did not appear to recognise that many girls wanted more than a practical training, a Hartnell uniform and a chance to work at Butlins! As schoolteachers pointed out on numerous occasions, girls of high academic ability needed intellectual stimulation; raising the standard of nurse entry requirements was of no use 'unless the course of training is geared to the intellectual ability of the trainee'.[71]

The expansion of female employment opportunities from 1945 onwards had attracted girls into hitherto predominantly male professions and it was therefore not realistic to expect intelligent girls to enter a nurse training school when they could just as easily enter medical school. Girls were also attracted to professions allied to medicine such as radiography, physiotherapy and occupational therapy, which offered patient contact without the imposition of archaic discipline. With the dropping of the marriage bar in most occupations and the continuing shortage of labour, girls were being wooed into employment spheres from all directions. As mobile recruitment vans toured the schools, nurses proclaiming the virtues of their profession were forced to compete with social workers, the police, airline companies and a wide assortment of industrial employers, all hoping to recruit children directly from school. The nursing profession remained 'firmly rooted in the nineteenth century'[72] and unable to compete with this array of career alternatives.

According to research conducted by the Briggs Committee, the numbers of new recruits did improve from 1965 onwards, despite the fact that numbers of 18-year-old girls continued to fall. However, this pattern was due to 'an increasing number of older entrants and to substantial intakes of immigrant nurses'.[73] GNC figures also indicated an improvement in student nurse wastage rates as demonstrated in Table 4.2 but, since these figures referred to selected groups, they do not present an accurate picture. The average student wastage rate over a period of three years was approximately 33%. This rate was lower than for women in general employment, but it was higher than the wastage rate for students in higher education, which included trainee teachers.[74] An analysis of hospital records also suggests that wastage rates varied markedly between regions and between individual hospitals within the same region. The wastage rate was higher than 50% in some hospitals while in others it was lower than 9%. Furthermore, these rates appeared to reflect the quality of training offered within individual nursing schools rather than variations in selection procedures. The overall situation, however, did not offer much comfort to ministers concerned with the restructuring of nurse administration.

Table 4.2 Annual percentage wastage rates of nurses (selected groups) in training in England and Wales, 1964/5-70/1a

	General		Mental		Mental Subnormality	
	Students	**Pupils**	**Students**	**Pupils**	**Students**	**Pupils**
1964/5	14.5	20.0	23.1		26.8	
1965/6	*11.8*	*20.4*	*19.4*	*18.6*	*21.3*	*33.3*
1966/7	13.0	20.0	20.5	43.7	22.7	35.8
1967/8	*12.7*	*22.6*	*19.0*	*34.4*	*21.9*	*25.1*
1968/9	12.3	19.8	18.5	25.0	19.1	21.9
1969/70	*11.3*	*19.2*	*17.0*	*23.8*	*18.0*	*12.9*
1970/1	10.0	18.2	14.1	17.8	16.7	17.8

Note: a Figures for students are annual rates of wastage from three-year courses as a percentage of the average number of nurses in training during the year (ending 31 March); for pupils, annual rates of wastage from two-year courses. A proportion of those who discontinue later return to nursing.
Source: Calculated from Reports of the General Nursing Council for England and Wales, annual.

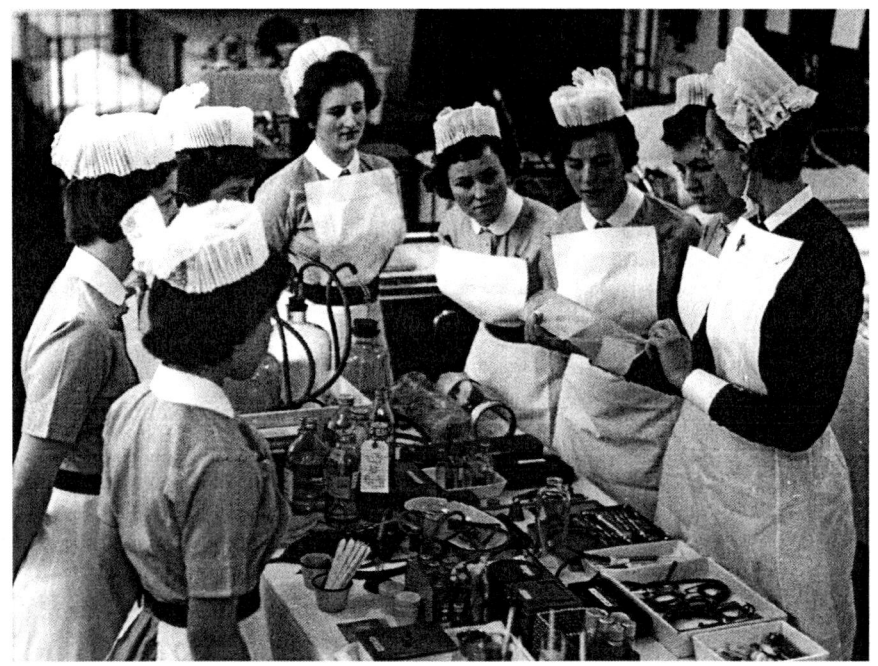

March 1960 - Student nurses in training at St Thomas's Hospital, London. Only 200 from every 2,000 applicants were accepted for training.

Endnotes

(1)   C. Webster, 'The nursing crises of the early National Health Service', *Bulletin of the History of Nursing Group,* 7 (1985), p.7
(2)   *Parliamentary Debates,*(House of Commons), 5th ser., 444, 20th November 1947, col.1333
(3)   Cohen, *op cit.,* p.9
(4)   Clay, *op cit.*
(5)   *British Nursing Journal,* September 1945, p.101
(6)   *Ibid.*
(7)   PRO DT/16/585. This one of the General Nursing Council files.
(8)   P. Howlett, *Fighting with the Figures* (1995)
(9)   PRO DT/16/585
(10)   Dame Elizabeth Cockayne, *op cit.*
(11)   PRO DT/16/585
(12)   Wood, *op cit.,* p.113
(13)   Dame Elizabeth Cockayne, *op cit.*
(14)   PRO DT/16/585
(15)   *Ibid.*
(16)   Warneford Hospital Archives RI/IF/1/1, Radcliffe Infirmary Nursing Minutes
(17)   Abel-Smith, *op cit.,* p.238-9
(18)   Wellcome Unit for the History of Medicine, Manchester, oral history transcripts of senior nurses working in the Manchester region during the 1960s; tape ref. N17/N18.
(19)   Clay, *op cit.,* p.118
(20)   PRO LAB/8/1388. This one of Ministry of Labour files which suggests guidelines for the employment of hospital staff
(21)   PRO MH/80/44. This one of Ministry of Health files regarding nurse recruitment
(22)   IWM/536/K16228
(23)   R.G.S. Brown and R.W.H. Stone, *The Male Nurse* (1973), p.17
(24)   *Parliamentary Debates (*House of Lords), 5th ser., 159, 9th November 1948, col.312
(25)   *Ibid.,* p.301
(26)   Brown and Stone, *op cit.,* p.20
(27)   *British Journal of Nursing,* editorial, November 1951
(28)   *Ibid.*
(29)   PRO MH55/ 2091. Correspondence pertaining to nurse recruitment problems
(30)   PRO LAB/8/1388 MH55/2091. Ministry of Health circular, MOH-94111/6/5
(31)   Royal London Hospital nursing minutes, 24th July 1950
(32)   Radcliffe Infirmary nursing minutes, 12th November 1952
(33)   Ministry of Health Cmd paper 9566, 31.12.54.
(34)   Brown and Stone, *op cit.,* p.21
(35)   Radcliffe Nursing advisory minutes RI/IF/1/1
(36)   PRO LAB/8/1388
(37)   *Ibid*
(38)   *Ibid.*
(39)   *British Journal of Nursing* editorial, February 1955
(40)   Wellcome Unit for the History of Medicine, Manchester. Oral history transcripts of senior nurses working in the Manchester region during the 1960s; tape N19.
(41)   PRO LAB/8/1388
(42)   R. Titmuss, *Essays On The Welfare State* (1958), p.102
(43)   Local authorities were not under any obligation to notify central government regarding decisions to withdraw nursery provision. Between 1st January and 31st March 1953 eighteen nurseries were closed. See *Parliamentary Debates* (House of Commons), 5th ser., 515, 14th May 1953, col.1385-1390. Following the closure of many nurseries in 1953 this policy was reversed in the 1960s to allow more women to enter full-time employment.
(44)   *Parliamentary Debates* (House of Commons), 5th ser., 732, 20th July 1966, col.754
(45)   Clay, *op cit.,* p.119
(46)   *Ibid.,* p.120
(47)   *Ibid.*

(48)   Baly, *op cit.*; unpublished paper given at the Royal College of Nursing, London. (1995), p.5

(49)   T. Kushner, 'An alien occupation', *Second Chance*, p.574

(50)   K. Lunn, 'Race and labour in Britain, 1850-1950', in K. Lunn, ed., *Race relations or industrial relations?* (1985), p.1-29

(51)   *Ibid.*

(52)   D. Bridges *A History of the International Council of Nurses* (1967)

(53)   *Parliamentary Debates,* (House of Lords), 5th ser., 159, 9th November 1948, col.1290

(54)   Kushner, *op cit.*, p. 575-6

(55)   Briggs, *op cit.*, p.122

(56)   Clay, *op cit.*, p.105

(57)   J Salvage *The Politics of Nursing* (1985), p.39

(58)   Cohen, *op cit.*, p.46

(59)   Wellcome Unit oral history transcript, tape N19

(60)   Briggs, *op cit.*, p.59

(61)   Salvage, *op cit.*, p.39

(62)   V. Chambers, 'Cadet schemes and their impact on the recruitment and wastage of student nurses', unpublished Ph.D. thesis, Manchester University, 1960, p.vi

(63)   Briggs, *op cit.*, p.117

(64)   PRO MH/55/2091. Ministry of Health files relating to nurse recruitment statistics

(65)   Chambers, *op cit.*, p.210

(66)   M. Baly, oral history transcript, interview conducted 7th November 1995

(67)   Chambers, *op cit.*, p.82

(68)   Chambers, *op cit.*, p.197

(69)   *Ibid.*, p.200

(70)   Briggs, *op cit.*, p.54

(71)   *Ibid.*

(72)   B. Salmon, oral history interview conducted October 1993

(73)   Briggs, *op cit.*, p.125

(74)   *Ibid.*, p.123

Chapter 5

Reasserting the Officer

From the late 1950s onwards the thrust of government policy with regard to the nursing profession shifted away from recruitment issues towards that of nurse administration. This move to restructure nurse administration was closely connected with government economic policy.

One of the most popular misconceptions relating to nursing issues and the emergence of the NHS has been the assumption that 'during the establishment of the regional hospital structure there was less concern with economy than with shortage of nurses'.[1] While recruitment difficulties undoubtedly dictated government policy towards the nursing profession, these difficulties were never allowed to entirely override economic considerations. From its inception, the NHS became a focus for political discontent, particularly with regard to the allocation of financial resources. The post-war Labour government was confronted with a precarious balance of payments deficit and an unexpected termination of the American lend-lease programme. This situation was compounded by the emergence of Cold War politics, which demanded a substantial increase in defence spending. Furthermore, although Britain managed to secure a new loan from America, the terms were restrictive and the interest payments crippling.

The government was thus forced to direct its economic policy towards increasing exports, which in turn required a substantial investment in the industrial sector. A policy of wage restraint was introduced and the Treasury was committed to curbing rises in expenditure within the social services and the NHS. It was not surprising, therefore, that concessions in the form of pay awards for nurses during this crucial period plunged the NHS into an economic crisis, since it was 'largely the nursing awards that led £392 million into becoming £400 million, the figure that was invoked for a decade as constituting the right cost for the NHS'.[2] An analysis of salary negotiations between government and nursing camps is provided in Chapter 8. The focus of the following analysis will concentrate on the issue of nursing administration because, within an increasingly unfavourable economic climate as Titmuss observed, there was a 'strong tendency to attribute all that is thought of as good or bad in medical care to a particular administrative structure and organisation'.[3] The Guilleband Report may have vindicated the NHS of gross extravagance but, within the realms of administration, the NHS was still regarded with some justification as costly and inefficient.

Government ministers had paid some attention to re-evaluating the system of nurse administration in the 1950s by attempting to apply industrial concepts to nursing organisation, but proposed changes outlined in the Goddard and Bradbeer reports were not implemented.[4] However, once the Conservative Government published its 'Hospital Plan' in 1962, administrative issues could no longer be kept on a political 'back burner'. The introduction of the 'Hospital Plan' was motivated by the need to integrate health services more fully and the structural framework relied on a system of grouping hospitals around a district general hospital, with the amalgamation of some psychiatric and general hospitals. This system of grouping required a professional administration programme to forge links between hospitals and to co-ordinate patient care. The 'Hospital Plan' was also designed to update the NHS and to accommodate the complex scientific advances that had been made in medical and nursing practice. As the Salmon Report acknowledged, 'new techniques are usually expensive and expert management will be needed, in which nurses should play their part, if costs are to be held in check'.[5] Researchers at Lancaster and Manchester Universities and the Institute for Operational Research had also suggested that nursing advisers should be incorporated into the management structure of hospital groups. Thus the issue of nurse administration became a dominant theme within the overall framework of the 'Hospital Plan'. Before discussing the administrative reforms that resulted from the publication of the Salmon Report in 1966, it is perhaps helpful to describe the administrative system prior to reform.

Nursing Administration Prior to the Implementation of Salmon

In 1948 the existing system of nurse administration was described by Dr Cohen as 'quasi-military in character' and, in addition to the strictly hierarchical structure, he argued that the regime was governed by the 'law of status'.[6] With the emergence of the NHS the system became more rather than less rigid, a process which was partly due to the scientific advances in medical practice. Medical technology demanded accuracy and discipline, therefore:

> ... *autocratic behaviour among hospital staffs, with behind them a long tradition deriving from military discipline, didactic teaching and poor law regimentation, is thereby strengthened by the invasion of scientific techniques, by increasing specialisation and by the growth of professional solidarities.*[7]

Significantly, this growth in the number and diversity of healthcare professionals had obscured the status of nursing, a process compounded by 'basic alterations to the chain of command'.[8]

General administration
The NHS had grouped hospitals together for administrative purposes, a process that had effectively excluded nurses from the decision-making process. Previously, matrons had been able to influence nursing policy in conjunction with medical superintendents or, in the case of voluntary hospitals, the board of governors. Regional Health Boards and Hospital Management Committees, however, did not include nurse representation and the position of the matron was severely undermined. By adopting a syndicalist approach, the medical profession had secured a dominant role in policy formulation, and White has rightly argued that the lack of nurse representation at group level undermined professional authority.[9] However, it is also clear that matrons were not equipped to adopt a more active role in policy formulation. The RCN had introduced administrative courses in preparation for the NHS, but these were restricted to a select few and they were not always relevant to current management procedures. Matrons generally viewed the prospect of committee meetings with a sense of trepidation, as Dame Kathleen Raven recalled, 'Even when they were asked to go to Hospital Management Committees they were reluctant to go. They were frightened'.[10]

Within hospitals
Furthermore, the role of the matron was ill-defined and differed between individual hospitals. Some matrons were responsible for radiography departments, for example, while others were excluded from this area of expertise altogether. There was also no discernible difference in status between matrons in charge of a small cottage hospital and those responsible for running a teaching hospital, except for salary differentials reflected in the Whitley scale according to bed occupancy. In psychiatric hospitals, the practice of employing a matron as head of the female nursing staff and a chief male nurse to supervise male nurses was clearly inefficient as administrative roles frequently overlapped. Decisions relating to nursing practice were made on an ad hoc basis and there was no attempt to incorporate forward planning procedures in relation to staff allocation or patient care. In addition, as the Salmon Committee noted:

As in industry and commerce where the belief survives that ability to manage is not learned but innate, nursing administration is still in the process of development. Few matrons appear to practise the technique of delegation. Nor do they seem to aim at decentralisation.[11]

Locally

The existing administrative structures also failed to provide effective communication networks between hospital and community nursing sectors. Patients were frequently discharged into the community without adequate nursing support, simply because district nurses had not been informed of their discharge. This problem was highlighted by the Conservative Minister of Health, Enoch Powell, at a RCN conference in 1963. During his address, Powell emphasised the need for improved co-ordination by means of a 'triangular circuit'; this circuit consisted of the general practitioner, the hospital and the local authority. Powell continued by stating that, 'If the vital information is to flow and there is to be no loss of contact at any point then a 'drill' is essential, under which responsibilities are precisely designed'.[12] Improved co-ordination of services, he argued, would result in a reduction of patient waiting lists and, in a further bid to tackle this problem, Powell also confirmed that he had 'asked regional boards to seek co-operation from the hospitals of the armed services'.[13]

Powell had stressed that the secret of good co-ordination lay with the 'placing of specific responsibility on designated individuals'[14] and the Salmon Committee investigating the structural framework of senior nursing staff appeared to endorse this view. Accordingly, the Salmon recommendations introduced clearly defined spheres of authority and combined them with management concepts. However, the introduction of a corporate model of organisation into a hitherto military hierarchy was fraught with difficulties. Since the Salmon structure was designed to create a nursing profession equal to that of the medical profession, the implementation of Salmon was considered by the latter group to be extremely controversial.

The Salmon Recommendations

Brian Salmon was first approached by the Ministry of Health in 1962 with a view to restructuring senior nursing staff, and the Committee began its investigations in 1963. Within a total membership of ten, the Committee included five nurses and, according to the Chairman, had no preconceived ideas regarding nursing organisation; the only nursing report consulted was the one compiled by the Bradbeer Committee in 1954. Bradbeer had suggested that, ideally, nurses should form a partnership with lay administrators and the medical profession. Predictably, this suggestion had not appealed to the medical profession, which expressed doubt as to the 'capability of nurses to assume roles other than resources to physicians'.[15] The Salmon Committee, however, did not share this doubt and argued that a systematic training programme in management skills would enable nurses to formulate policy within the hospital staffing structure, both at a local and regional level. At a national level, senior nurses at Whitehall already exerted considerable influence on government policy through the Standing Nursing Advisory Committee and via their own nursing division.

The acquisition of management skills, however, was not in itself enough to assert the nursing position within the NHS; a new strategic staffing structure was necessary to assist managerial functions. A pyramid structure was therefore proposed and senior nurses were allocated positions in top, middle and first-line management. Spheres of influence were divided into divisions, sections and units, and senior nurses were given the title 'Officer'. Within the Salmon system, the function of top management was to formulate nursing policy and to apply it within a division. Middle management was responsible for programming nursing policy within a specified unit and first-line management for executing policy within a section. The basic concept was to 'bring together work in which the decisions are appropriate to a given level of management and to constitute jobs accordingly'.[16] (Diagrams demonstrating the application of the Salmon structure are included at the end of this chapter; source: Salmon Report, 1966.)

The report also suggested that the aims of nursing policy should be directed towards providing a high standard of nursing care and evaluating professional training requirements, and that:

> ... the patient himself should be seen, however, as fighting in the front line of the battle against illness - with the nursing, medical and other staff together providing the forward support, the intelligence and weapons and the vital supplies. [17]

Nurses may not have viewed their role in precisely the same terms as the Salmon Report, but they did warm to the military flavour of the structure since the introduction of divisions, units and sections, combined with the Officer title, appealed to their sense of military tradition.

The restructuring of senior nursing staff into top, middle and first-line management also held significant financial implications, albeit that salary considerations were outside the remit of the Salmon enquiry. Whereas, prior to Salmon, a matron in a small hospital was accorded the same title as a matron in a teaching hospital, following reforms the matron of the smaller hospital was relegated to middle management. This practice of according lower status to nurses in charge of smaller establishments had, in fact, been in operation within military circles before the Second World War, where small hospitals were run by a senior sister rather than a matron. Ostensibly, this practice was implemented by the military to allow senior nurses to gain administrative experience. However, in reality it was a thinly disguised cost-cutting exercise.

Similarly, the implications of how posts were graded within the Salmon structure, and the remuneration for such posts, gave the government cause for concern. Previously, salaries had been determined by the number of hospital beds and the existence of nurse training schools. However, this criterion for determining salaries was not particularly reliable as, Salmon argued:

> *Numbers of beds in themselves do not make a job more difficult and the need to co-ordinate the requirements of nurse training and nursing service is only one factor among many; others are the complexities of nursing administration in a teaching hospital, the different kinds of nurse training courses administered, the numbers of students and pupils, the busyness of wards and clinics as measured by turnover and attendances, and the kinds of specialist unit.* [18]

The report argued, therefore, that remuneration should be based on the 'quality of decisions to be taken and the relative difficulty of jobs falling within the same grades'.[19] Ministers, however, argued that the issue of remuneration was already problematic since nurses had been protesting against the Treasury policy of wage restraint for some time. Moreover, the government, which had originally initiated the Salmon enquiry, was replaced by the Wilson administration in 1964. When the Salmon Report was published in 1966, Britain was experiencing a sterling crisis and an increasing amount of industrial unrest. Furthermore, as nurses exerted pressure on the government with the RCN's 'Raise the Roof' campaign, pay demands threatened to destroy the Prices and Incomes Policy. For this reason alone, the timing of administrative reforms adopted a political significance and, as Brian Salmon recalled:

> *The nursing department at the Ministry of Health was overruled by politicians over the timing of the new management structure - and it was all because the Secretary of State had agreed salary increases for nurses which they decided to implement based on Salmon.* [20]

By implementing the reforms in conjunction with new salary scales, the government had hoped to convince the electorate that nurses were a special case. Concessions to nurses, they argued, did not therefore signal an end to wage restraint in other employment sectors.

The Implementation of Salmon

Following the publication of the Salmon Report in 1966, a leading article in the *Nursing Mirror* proclaimed that 'it need not be long before the Salmon structure could be in full swing and the present rigid authoritarian system merely a hideous memory'.[21] Despite this display of optimism on the part of professional bodies, the implementation of Salmon was far from straightforward. Although recruitment figures had substantially improved due to the influx of immigrant nurses, the majority of these had qualified as second-grade nurses and were unable to perform administrative tasks. Even if registered nurses had existed in greater numbers, they were not by the nature of their training equipped for administrative posts and, as previously acknowledged, administrative reforms had for some time been constrained by a lack of trained nurses with administrative experience (see Table 5.1). Existing training programmes in nurse administration were few and far between and generally of a poor quality. In addition, many nurses had adopted a similar attitude to the field of administration as they had to that of education, and had argued that clinical nursing should take precedence over both these fields.

Salmon attempted to resolve this problem by creating managerial posts that still required some clinical expertise. The structural changes also included a promotional pathway which, in theory at least, allowed nurses working in clinical areas the same opportunities for advancement as those working in the areas of management and education. However, the success of the Salmon proposals relied heavily on the adequate preparation of nurses for management roles, and a clear acknowledgement from within the profession of the levels of nursing expertise. Such acknowledgement was not forthcoming. Instead there was considerable confusion and bitter wrangling, not only with regard to nursing expertise but also with regard to the boundaries of authority imposed by the Salmon reforms. The subtle nuances associated with management techniques were lost on nurses. The Salmon system did provide clear guidelines for spheres of nursing influence but these clashed with the traditional military model of administration. For instance, a senior night nursing officer was considered by Salmon to be 'in charge' whereas other senior nursing officers were defined as being 'in control'. In reality this terminology merely reflected the difference between those nurses who had overall control and determination of policy and those who assumed periodic control. Nurses, however, were used to being in charge and having control simultaneously! There were also particular problems associated with the Principal Nursing Officer (teaching)

Table 5.1
Number of staff who had undertaken certain administrative courses

Grade	Number of staff	Administrative qualifications					
		A	B	C	D	E	F
A. England and Wales							
All staff	37,393	12	277	98	141	372	227
Matron (women)	*1,835*	*1*	*109*	*40*	*5*	*8*	*42*
Matron /chief male nurse (men)	210	—	1	—	—	—	—
Deputy etc. matron (women)	*2,469*	*4*	*106*	*47*	*5*	*2*	*4*
Deputy, matron, chief, male nurse (men)	*904*	*1*	*10*	—	*6*	*3*	*6*
Midwifery tutorial staff	*236*	*1*	*2*	*1*	*1*	*1*	*4*
Nursing tutorial staff (women)	1,022	2	12	—	7	22	84
Nursing tutorial staff (men)	*412*	—	—	—	*1*	—	*17*
Departmental midwifery sister	281	—	1	—	—	1	—
Departmental sister	*2,191*	—	*25*	*8*	*9*	*32*	*8*
Departmental charge nurse	153	—	—	—	2	—	—
Midwifery sister	*3,247*	—	—	—	—	*13*	—
Ward sister	15,766	3	6	1	93	221	23
Charge nurse	*5,251*	—	—	—	*5*	*6*	*12*
Other senior midwifery staff	203	—	2	—	—	—	—
Other senior nursing staff (women)	*2,851*	—	*3*	*1*	*5*	*23*	*9*
Other senior nursing staff (men)	362	—	—	—	2	1	3
B. Scotland							
All staff	4,802	2	55	—	118	7	—
Matron (women)	*284*	—	*17*	—	*1*	*1*	*16*
Matron / chief male nurse (men)	14	—	—	—	—	—	1
Deputy etc. matron (women)	*290*	—	*23*	—	*4*	*3*	—
Deputy, matron, chief, male nurse (men)	90	—	4	—	2	—	3
Midwifery tutorial staff	*36*	*1*	—	—	—	—	—
Nursing tutorial staff (women)	131	1	—	—	4	—	7
Nursing tutorial staff (men)	*50*	—	—	—	—	—	—
Departmental midwifery sister	36	—	—	—	1	—	—
Departmental sister	*201*	—	*7*	—	*5*	—	—
Departmental charge nurse	6	—	—	—	1	—	—
Midwifery sister	*501*	—	—	—	—	—	—
Ward sister	2,331	—	3	—	90	3	3
Charge nurse	*516*	—	—	—	*9*	—	—
Other senior midwifery staff	18	—	—	—	—	—	—
Other senior nursing staff (women)	*274*	—	—	—	*1*	—	—
Other senior nursing staff (men)	24	—	1	—	—	—	—

Key:
A = Diploma in Nursing Administration (University of Edinburgh);
B = Administrative Certificate of RCN;
C = One-year administrative course at King Edward's Fund Staff College;
D = Ward Sister's Certificate of RCN;
E = Three months Ward Sister's Course at King Edward's Fund Staff College;
F = Diploma in Nursing.
Source: Salmon Report (1966).

and the Principal Nursing Officer (nursing). The management side of the Whitley Council maintained that the PNO of a teaching division was responsible for preparing a practical plan of teaching, whereas the staff side argued that this responsibility lay with the PNO of a nursing division. This confusion was used later by the Whitley Council to delay nurse pay awards. But the major problem associated with the implementation of Salmon lay with an ongoing reluctance on the part of the government to provide an adequate number of appropriate management courses for nurses. This required government funding, and such investment was not forthcoming.

The ensuing chaos within nurse administration was predictable. The Ministry of Health had been advised by hospital representatives prior to the Salmon reforms that this lack of investment in nurse management courses would subsequently distort the implementation of the Salmon system and cause administrative chaos. A letter written to the Ministry of Health from the Royal London Hospital, for instance, stated that 'it would seem unfortunate if, through undue haste, these hospitals without the necessary finance or personnel should implement a Salmon-type structure and yet be unable to conform to the underlying principles'.[22] Nevertheless, when the Salmon system was finally implemented from 1969 onwards, such warnings were ignored. As Brian Salmon recalled, 'With the exception of a handful of pilot schemes, nurses were already in post and just assumed new titles without any preparation for their new management roles'.[23]

Due to inept government handling, therefore, Salmon reforms merely reinforced an old regime. Senior nurses were unable to adapt to their new roles since they found it difficult to grasp management concepts without appropriate training. Indeed, 'their educational limitations left them cruelly exposed'.[24] In effect, senior nurses were given more power but not the skills to wield it. Rank and file nurses were also confused by administrative reforms; under the previous system the matron had in theory supported the welfare of her nurses, but within the new system senior nurses were expected to support the management line in policy decisions and, in this respect, Salmon was divisive. However, the fundamental problem lay with the fact that senior nurses were still '"officers", not managers, a leftover from a bygone age and they did not even command the support of their troops'.[25] The lack of an adequate knowledge base in management skills also fostered a level of professional insecurity and, as a result, nurses were more, rather than less, reluctant to relinquish their traditional hierarchy. As Salvage has noted, the senior nurses who adhered rigidly to the hierarchy as a means of security were the same people who espoused the cause of professionalism. They failed to see 'the contradiction in their position; a true professional who is an independent practitioner accountable to patients and peers for her practice has no need of any army style structure to keep her in line'.[26]

Nevertheless, although the Salmon system did little to change the notion of hierarchy, it did have the effect of encouraging more men into the profession. The proliferation of non-clinical posts that accompanied administrative reforms allowed for quicker promotion in a variety of areas. Prior to Salmon, men were generally not promoted until the age of forty and the exclusionary practices exerted by female nurses had considerably narrowed their promotional field. There was a certain sense of irony, therefore, in that these exclusionary practices had also ensured that men were better placed than women to take advantage of the Salmon reforms. Within the new promotional structure, career advancement was concentrated in the areas of nurse management and education. As previously acknowledged, men had opted for careers in nurse education because they were frequently denied promotion in the area of clinical practice. With the implementation of Salmon, therefore, men discovered that, in terms of promotional opportunities, they were in a strong strategic position. The failure of women to provide support networks for their own sex to counteract this position resulted in a male takeover of senior nursing posts.

While Salmon provided a stimulus to the recruitment of male nurses, the reforms did not achieve an efficient administrative system. This in itself was not surprising as nurse administration had been dealt with in isolation. The overall administrative system within the health service was totally out of touch with modern management techniques, and there was no real logic in reorganising nurse administration without also reorganising all the administration pertaining to healthcare delivery. Undoubtedly the problem of introducing efficient administrative systems into the health service formed part of a wider debate that centred on the concept of corporate management versus the supposed altruistic nature of the welfare state. As Cohen had argued in 1948, the nursing role in healthcare both in the curative and preventive fields could be viewed as 'a form of industry as well as a public service, rather like industry proper in the nationalised sectors. We may therefore use nursing criteria of efficiency developed in industry'.[27] This view, however, did not find favour with healthcare professionals who considered the NHS as being far removed from industrial concerns and that patients were endangered by the fact that 'the ends or aims of hospital work may be obscured by excessive preoccupation with means'.[28]

The role of government within this debate was to try and reconcile the need to curb NHS spending while simultaneously providing adequate standards of patient care. But since no formula existed for measuring the standards of patient care, nor for measuring medical or administrative efficiency, government policy was usually incoherent, ill-advised and at times completely incompetent.

Amid the confusion, nurses relied heavily on routine and tradition,[29] rejecting corporate management not for the concept of altruism but for the safe confines of military hierarchy.

Conclusion

Government policy had attempted to influence nurse administration, but this influence in most instances made little or no impact on the military traditions and customs of the nursing profession. Since the demobilisation of service personnel had coincided with the emergence of the NHS, the long-standing military influence within civilian nursing was reinforced. Consequently, there was always the danger, as Titmuss had pointed out, that, 'a new authoritarianism will replace or be superimposed on the old one'.[30] This prediction materialised in the guise of the Salmon reforms. As Brian Salmon recalled, 'the military imposition in the form of the Nightingale legacy was still very much alive in the middle of the 1960s'.[31] This military legacy had been reinforced since Nightingale by two world wars and was strengthened by a concept of military efficiency. Nurses remained overly concerned with their status and the government preoccupied with recruitment; consequently, there was no attempt to 'protect the patient and avoid placing him or her in the no-mans-land between the trenches'. Whereas government attempts to influence nurse recruitment had met with limited success, the administrative reforms were an unmitigated disaster.[32] As Salmon himself stated, the implementation of his report of 1966 proved to be a 'real catastrophe'. The corporate model of organisation had challenged the military model, and the latter had withstood the challenge.

Application of the Salmon Structure -Chart 1
ST DOMINICS HOSPITAL BOARD OF GOVERNORS
St. Dominics is a teaching hospital on a single site

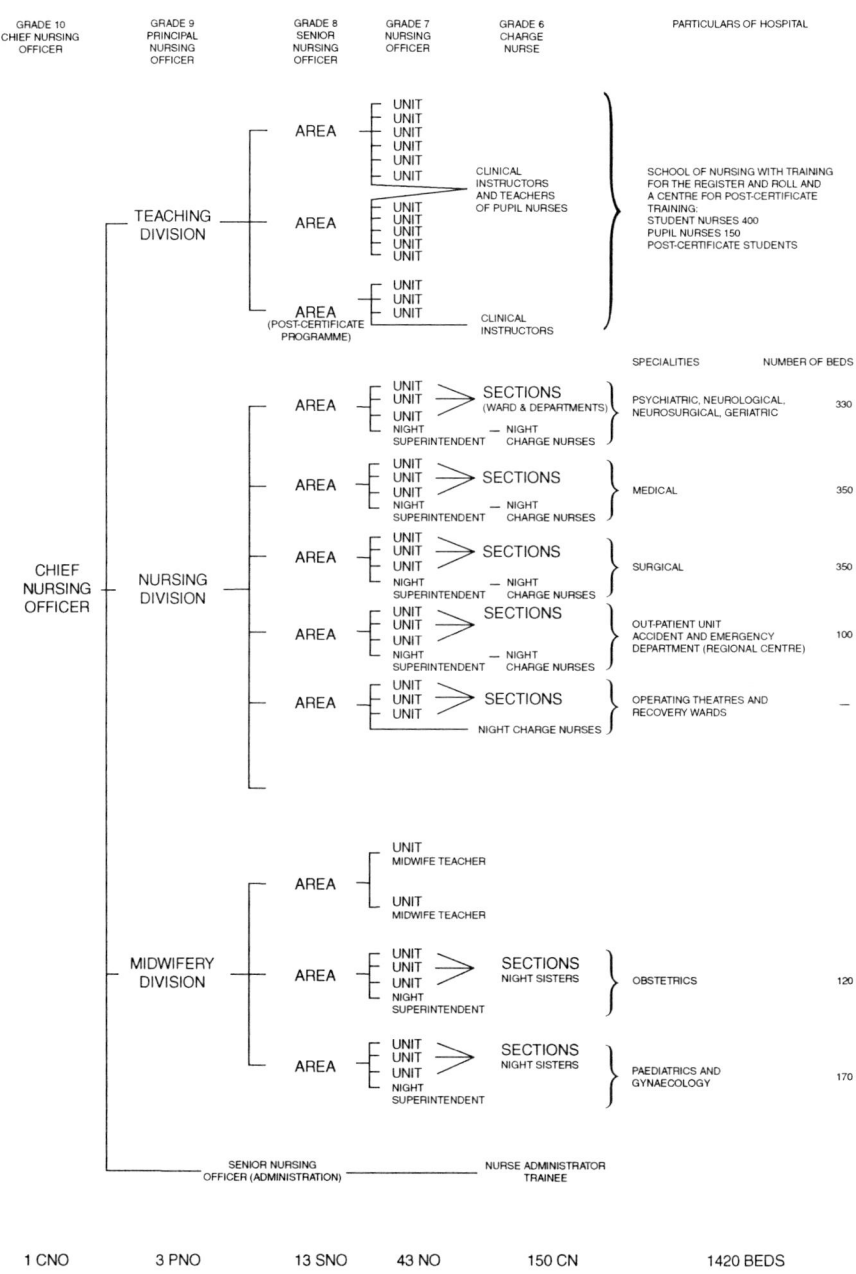

Application of the Salmon Structure -Chart 2

WESTERN HOSPITAL MANAGEMENT COMMITTEE

This group consists of a single mental illness hospital with 1500 beds. The nursing service is controlled by a Chief Male Nurse (category (a)) and a Matron, on the male and female sides respectively. The hospital has a Medical Superintendent.

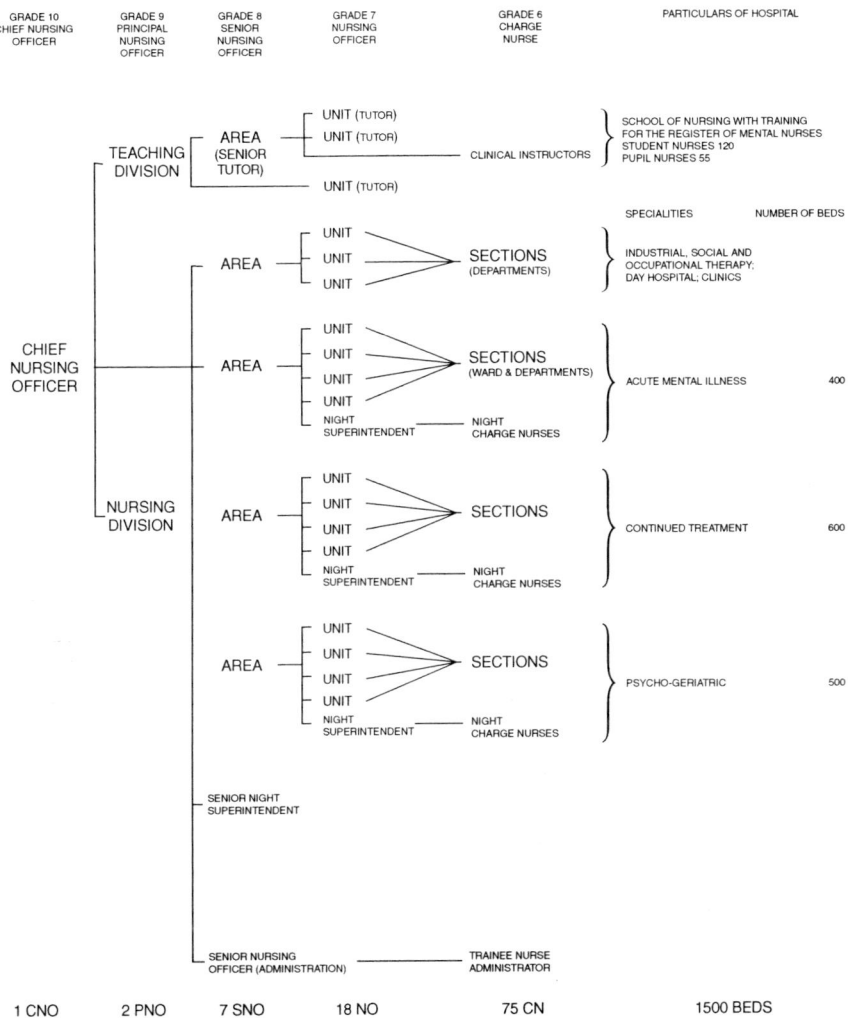

GRADE 10 CHIEF NURSING OFFICER	GRADE 9 PRINCIPAL NURSING OFFICER	GRADE 8 SENIOR NURSING OFFICER	GRADE 7 NURSING OFFICER	GRADE 6 CHARGE NURSE	PARTICULARS OF HOSPITAL

1 CNO	2 PNO	7 SNO	18 NO	75 CN	1500 BEDS

Application of the Salmon Structure -Chart 3

NORTH MANFORD AND DISTRICT H.M.C.

The group has seven hospitals with a total of 2,295 beds. Nearly half the beds are in the two branches of North Manford Hospital and nearly a third in a Whitestone Hospital. The hospitals are in five different places, which is reflected in the present nursing administration. The mental illness hospital is at one centre (13 miles from North Manford Hospital) and has a Matron and a Chief Male Nurse. The other six hospitals are in four centres with a Matron at each centre: North Manford; Greencroft; Thornywood and Mapleton Hospitals (close to each other and about 10 miles from North Manford); Westwood Maternity Hospital (6 miles from North Manford); and Northern Hospital (13 miles from North Manford). There are five hospital secretaries in the group - one to each centre. All the hospitals, except Northern and Westwood Maternity Hospitals, have Medical Superintendents and North Manford has one at each branch.

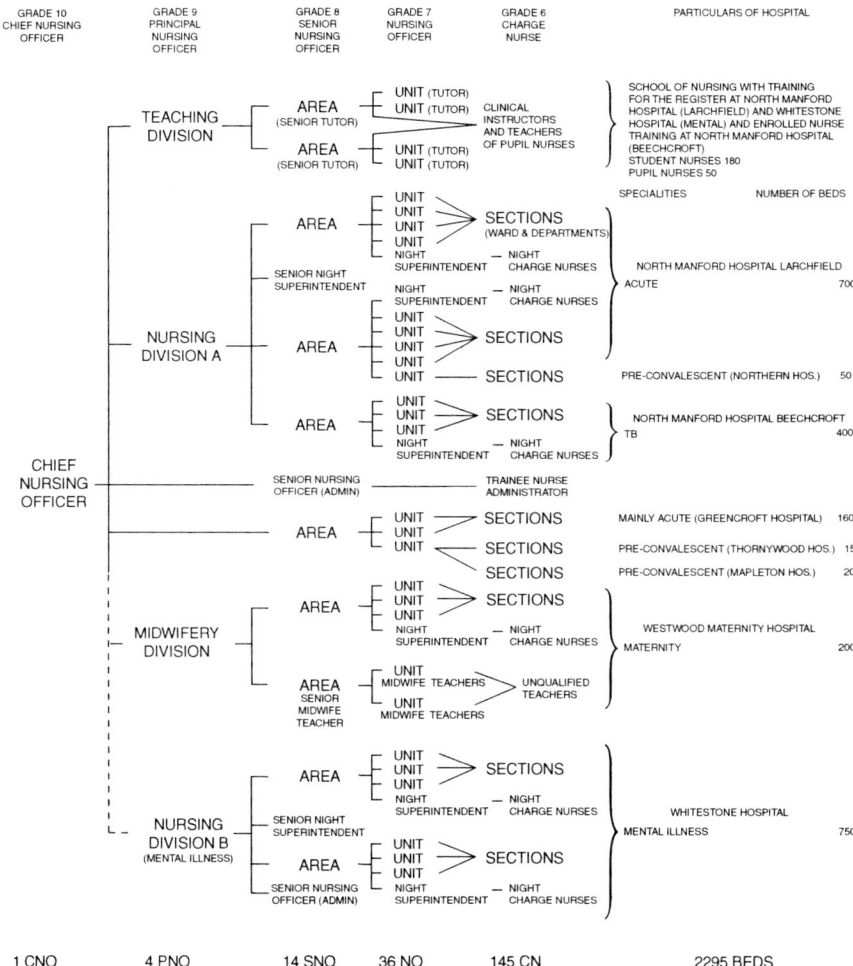

Application of the Salmon Structure -Chart 4

BARCHESTER AND DISTRICT H.M.C.

The group has 1,700 beds in fourteen hospitals - seven General, three small Maternity, two Chronic Sick, one Chest Hospital and a Convalescent Home. Eight of the hospitals (with seven independent nursing heads) are in three main population centres, within 10 miles of each other and each with a large General Hospital. The other six hospitals (each with independent nursing heads) are dispersed - up to 15 miles away. There are nine Hospital Secretaries and the administrative headquarters are at the Crosse Street branch of the Barchester Royal Infirmary.

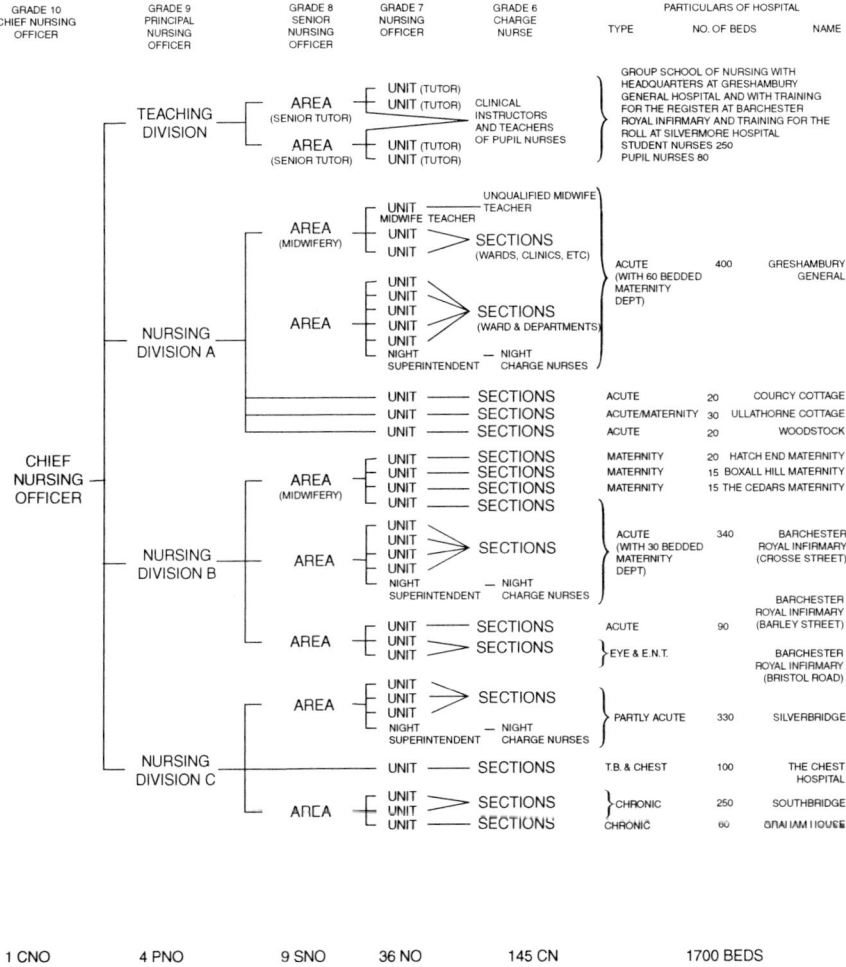

GRADE 10 CHIEF NURSING OFFICER	GRADE 9 PRINCIPAL NURSING OFFICER	GRADE 8 SENIOR NURSING OFFICER	GRADE 7 NURSING OFFICER	GRADE 6 CHARGE NURSE	PARTICULARS OF HOSPITAL

1 CNO	4 PNO	9 SNO	36 NO	145 CN	1700 BEDS

Application of the Salmon Structure -Chart 5

GRESHAMBURY & ULLATHORNE
HOSPITAL MANAGEMENT COMMITTEE

This group consists of two mental illness hospitals and a mental subnormality hospital, each with its own Matron and Chief Male Nurse. Greshambury House (mental subnormality, 1500 beds) is adjacent to Manor House (mental illness, 200 beds). Ullathorne Park (mental illness, 600 beds) is three miles away. Greshambury House and Manor House each have their own Physician Superintendent. Each hospital has its own Hospital Secretary, who in the case of Ullathorne Park is also the Group Secretary.

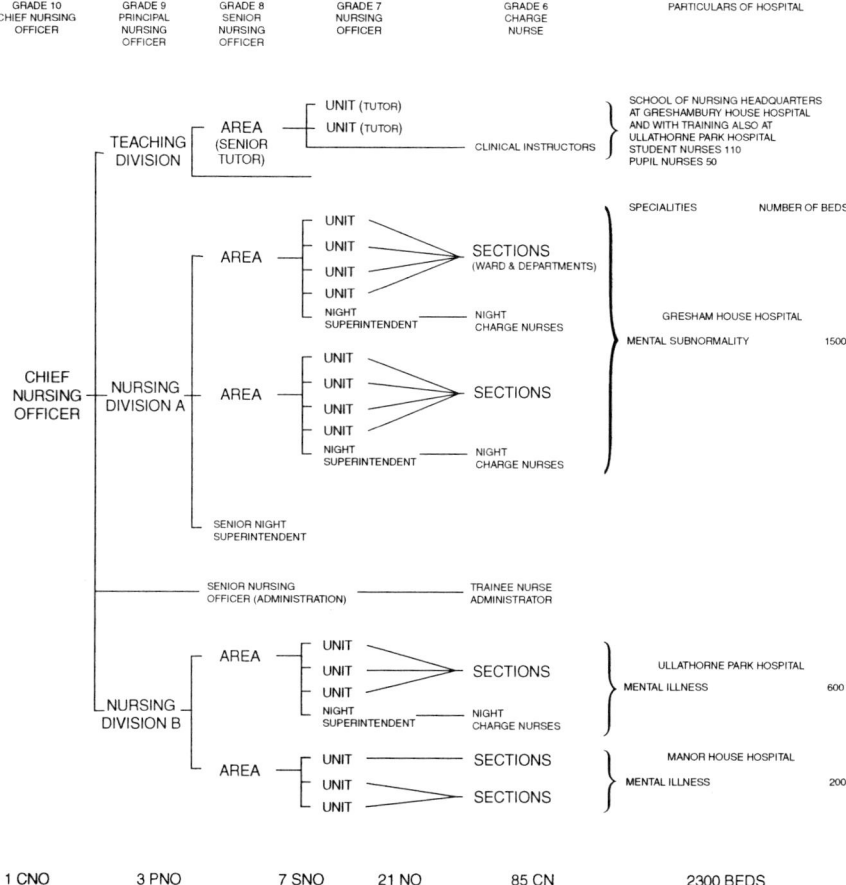

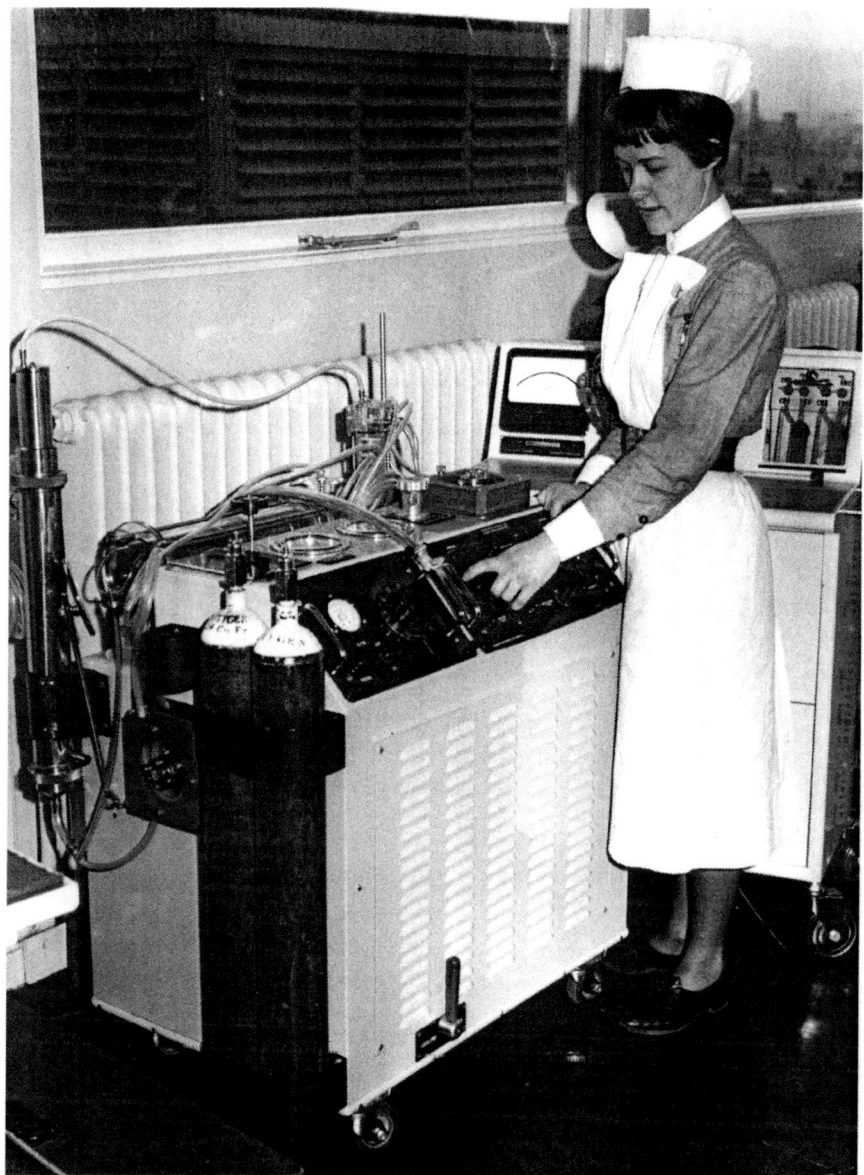

January 1962 - One of the first artificial heart machines is introduced at The Royal Infirmary, Sheffield. The machine cost £10,000.

Endnotes

(1)   C. Webster, 'The nursing crisis of the early National Health Service', *Bulletin of the History of Nursing Group*, 7 (1985), p.7

(2)   Webster, *op cit.*, p.9

(3)   R. Titmuss, *op. cit.*, p.184

(4)   Goddard Report published in 1953; Bradbeer Report published in 1954.
The Goddard Report was the result of a joint initiative by the Minister of Health and the Nuffield Provincial Hospitals Trust and provided a job analysis supervised by Mr H.A. Goddard, Chairman of the management side of the Whitley Council for Nurses and Midwives. The report was viewed as an attempt to apply industrial concepts to nursing practice and organisation. The report recommended teamwork, the formation of nursing units and a less hierarchical structure.

(5)   Salmon, *op cit.*, p.19

(6)   Cohen, *op cit.*, p.47

(7)   Titmuss, *op cit.*, p.201

(8)   White, *op cit.*, p.148

(9)   *Ibid.*, p.61

(10)   RCNA RCN/13/ED/1. Dame Kathleen Raven oral history transcript, March 1988

(11)   Salmon, *op cit.*, p.4

(12)   RCNA RCN/10/29. Address by Enoch Powell to the Royal College of Nursing Conference in 1963

(13)   *Ibid.*

(14)   *Ibid.*

(15)   R. and V. Splane, *Chief Nursing Officer Positions in National Ministries of Health* (University of California Press, 1995), p.124

(16)   Salmon, *op cit.*, p.25

(17)   *Ibid.*

(18)   Salmon, *op cit.*, p.28

(19)   *Ibid.*, p.27

(20)   Salmon, letter to author dated 12 June 1995

(21)   *The Nursing Mirror*, 122 no. 7 (1966), p.125

(22)   Royal London Hospital Nursing Advisory Minutes, 1st October 1968

(23)   Salmon, oral history interview conducted October 1993

(24)   C. Hart, *Behind the Mask* (1994), p.188

(25)   *Ibid.*, p.189

(26)   Salvage, *op cit.*, p.85

(27)   Cohen, *op cit.*, p.35

(28)   Titmuss, *op cit.*, p.121

(29)   Clay, *op cit.*, p.102

(30)   R. Titmuss, *op. cit.*, p.201

(31)   Salmon, oral history interview conducted in October 1993

(32)   Clay, *op cit.*, p.2

Chapter 6

Masters of their Profession
or Slaves to the System?
Nurse Leadership and Nursing Practice

Although government officials had recognised that the nursing profession was, in reality, a mass of inconsistencies, policy initiatives were not designed to resolve this problem. Ministers argued that the responsibility for ironing out these inconsistencies and for dictating the scope and direction of nursing development lay strictly with the profession itself. It was abundantly clear, however, that in 1948 the nursing profession was ill-equipped to construct a cohesive nursing service and demonstrated an overwhelming reluctance to initiate changes in nursing development. According to White, professional stagnation was due primarily to a lack of nurse leaders,[1] but this assessment of the situation is fundamentally flawed since White's analysis fails to examine the relationship between rank and file nurses and their leaders, and makes no allowances for differing levels of leadership. As the following analysis will reveal, nurses' perception of their professional leadership and actual leadership were not one and the same.

However, although nurse leaders existed, did they have the power to prevent this stagnation? In order to initiate change nurses needed to be influential in policy formulation both at national and local level. As Haywood and Hunter have argued, the power relationships affecting healthcare policy were based on 'iron triangles' that consisted of civil servants, ministers and doctors.[2] According to Hart, unless nurses were able to break this triangle they could not 'seriously challenge the dominant position of the medical profession'.[3] But it can be argued that nurses were in the grip of another iron triangle, formed by military influence, religious beliefs and royal patronage. This latter triangle provided a greater obstacle to change than the former.

The problems that accompanied professional development significantly affected patient care. Overt identification with military culture and values reinforced the nursing hierarchy and increased regimentation in nursing practice. Whereas the medical hierarchy ultimately depended upon tacit understanding, the nursing hierarchy relied on 'a system of ranks and job specification'.[4] The degree of regimentation in nursing practice before the war had reached ludicrous proportions in several hospitals and 'ward sisters came on duty to an immaculate ward, every patient's nose in line with the centre crease of the top sheet'.[5] With the emphasis on post-war military efficiency, regimentation in nursing practice did not begin to subside until the late 1960s.

Nevertheless, regardless of nursing influence, changes in nursing practice were largely dictated by advances in medical technology.[6] In this sense nursing policy became reactive rather than pre-emptive, and scientific advance often served to increase rather than decrease existing regimentation. As Titmuss observed, the complexity of new surgical and medical procedures, and the timing and co-ordination of treatments, demanded new rules and regulations. Thus 'autocratic behaviour among hospital staffs' was 'strengthened by the invasion of scientific techniques, by increasing specialisation and by the growth of professional solidarities'.[7]

Nurses themselves could not decide whether nursing was an 'art' or a 'science' and hotly debated the merits and drawbacks of authoritarian regimes. Establishing professional boundaries between nurses and other healthcare workers was also problematic.[8] These issues were confronted by strong dynamic nurse leaders, but these same leaders failed consistently to gain the support of rank and file nurses.[9] Constraints on nursing development therefore were self-imposed rather than the result of external forces.

Nursing Leadership

Throughout the summer of 1948, the national and nursing press were in no doubt as to the identity of Britain's nurse leader. Dame Louisa Wilkinson, Matron in Chief of Queen Alexandra's Imperial Military Nursing Service and newly elected President of the Royal College of Nursing (RCN), was, according to press reports, 'Britain's most important nurse'.[10] Dame Louisa was pictured in full military regalia leading a procession of two hundred nurses to St Margaret's Church, Westminster, for the service that traditionally preceded the RCN annual conference. The four-day event was held between 30th June and 3rd July and, in view of the impending NHS reforms, it might be assumed that these would dominate conference proceedings. Potentially, the gathering of senior nurses offered the opportunity to discuss future strategies for patient care, to outline possible aims and objectives regarding nurse education and to consider the nursing skills which may be required to cope with new medical techniques such as blood transfusion. Instead, the conference was entitled 'The Nurses in the Social Order'[11] and topics for discussion reflected the profession's continuing obsession with status. Prominent speakers consisted primarily of London hospital matrons and the former editor of the *Nursing Times*. While Aneurin Bevan attended the conference, his speech was merely designed to reassure nurses that compulsory direction of labour would not be a feature of the new NHS. Despite all the pomp and ceremony, the conference agenda did not confront major nursing issues.

If rank and file nurses had expected changes in professional policy to emerge from this auspicious gathering of head nurses, they were destined for disappointment. The conference reaffirmed the nurses' place in the social order, but failed to give any clear indication of professional direction. There appeared to be a sense of complacency amongst conference participants and a pervading attitude that the existing British nursing service was the best in the world. But in view of the forthcoming changes in healthcare delivery, why did the President of the RCN as head of 47,000 nurses adopt such a complacent attitude? More importantly, why did the rank and file accept such complacency? Was their identification and perception of nurse leadership distorted? If press reports had wrongly identified 'Britain's most important nurse' then who, if anyone, could justifiably lay claim to this title? What were their priorities in terms of professional development? In order to answer these questions it is necessary in the first instance to determine the degree of professional and political influence exerted by nurse leaders and to assess their aims and objectives. Following on from this assessment, the analysis will explore the professional expectations of rank and file nurses.

Levels of Leadership

Prior to 1941 the strands of nurse leadership appeared to be relatively straightforward. Leaders within professional organisations such as the RCN represented general nurses while the leaders of unions such as the Mental Hospital and Institutional Workers Union (MHIWU) represented mental nurses. The formation of a nursing division within the Ministry of Health in 1941, however, heralded the arrival of a new and elevated level of leadership. As acknowledged in previous chapters, in addition to the Chief Nursing Officer (CNO) position at the Ministry of Health, senior nursing appointments were also established at the Ministry of Labour and National Service and at the Colonial Office. In terms of political leverage, nurses working at Whitehall were potentially able to influence government policy to a far greater extent than representatives of various nursing groups.

Despite this potential, these nurses, according to White, made little impact on policy formulation since the:

> *... nursing officers at the Ministry were a small group and were*
> *advisory rather than executive; and if civil servants felt disdain*

for nurses, they probably tended to disregard the advice given by these nurses. [12]

However, analysis of committee reports and official documents suggests that senior nurses at the Ministry significantly influenced policy direction and there was no indication that civil servants viewed nurses with any greater or lesser disdain than other occupational groups. On the contrary, the Ministry appeared to welcome nursing advice and senior nurses were afforded considerable levels of autonomy. As Dame Elizabeth Cockayne, CNO at the Ministry of Health in 1945, recalled:

The terms of reference given to her by the Chief Medical Officer to whom she was responsible consisted of the phrase 'just do as you think best'. [13]

Dame Kathleen Raven, who assumed the role of CNO in 1958, even managed to extricate herself totally from the supervision of the Medical Officer. This move resulted in greater autonomy for the nursing division as a whole. Logically, therefore, the level of nurse participation in policy formulation should form the major criteria for assessing actual rather than perceived nurse leadership. On this basis, evidence confirms that 'Britain's most important nurse' was in reality the CNO at Whitehall and not the President of the RCN. Rank and file nurses, however, appeared to be oblivious to this fact and viewed leadership in terms of the RCN President and the Association of Hospital Matrons (AHM). Meanwhile, by 1948 mental health nurses had merged union membership of the MHIWU with the Hospital and Welfare Services Union, forming the Confederation of Health Service Employees (COHSE). Significantly both the RCN and COHSE experienced leadership problems and neither group fully appreciated the leadership offered by nurses within the Ministry of Health. Herein lay the crux of the problem - nurses continued to follow their perceived leadership while simultaneously alienating their actual leadership.

Nurses at Whitehall

Dame Elizabeth Cockayne assumed the role of CNO at the Ministry of Health four months before the official inauguration of the NHS and was given a 'free hand' with regard to nursing development. Liaison networks were established, incorporating nursing officers and public health nursing officers from each of the fourteen Regional Health Authorities,[14] and policy was formulated at the centre through the Standing Nursing Advisory Committee (SNAC). The SNAC was one of a number of specialist committees included in the Central Health Services Council (CHSC) advisory machinery, which assisted the Minister of

Health in all matters affecting healthcare services. The CHSC membership was dominated by the medical profession and White has assumed, therefore, that nursing influence within this body was minimal.[15] According to Dame Elizabeth, however, it was possible to exert considerable influence through the Chairman of the CHSC[16] and through direct contact with the Minister of Health. Apparently, sporadic tension arose between senior nurses and civil servants as the latter group 'didn't like being excluded' from policy decisions,[17] but in a general sense it was relatively easy to promote nursing issues.

Significantly, however, the mere existence of such tension indicated that senior nurses were able to initiate and develop policy statements to a far greater degree than has previously been recognised. It was also clear that nurses at Whitehall were fighting a two-fronted battle: the first, with politicians and members of the medical profession, was to ensure that nursing issues remained high on the political agenda; the second was with members of their own profession, who needed to be convinced that nursing reforms were necessary in order to achieve real progress. While some doctors were supportive of nursing concerns, 'the medical profession as a whole were not'.[18] Many doctors accused nurses of inefficiency and viewed them as subordinates rather than as colleagues. Nurses were not the only group of healthcare workers to be labelled inefficient. A senior orthopaedic consultant claimed that physiotherapists were extremely inefficient, like 'butterflies flitting in and out of hospital wards and quite useless'. He further stated that the Health Service was 'overpopulated with such species'.[19] General practitioners were also despised by consultants.

Not all nurses and healthcare professionals were efficient but, since there were no satisfactory means of testing efficiency levels, it was difficult to prove the extent of existing inefficiency. Furthermore, the CHSC itself could not claim to be efficient since it had no set objectives and responded to healthcare issues in an ad hoc fashion. The Council attempted to develop policy statements 'but it was a time of change and they had to take each day as it came. They made decisions on the hoof'.[20] Over a period of time the situation improved and, despite economic constraints, by the mid 1950s healthcare planning began to adopt a sense of direction, particularly in the field of mental health. Senior nurses were able to promote nursing issues within healthcare planning, but there was very little evidence to suggest that policies were well received at hospital and community level. Indeed, it was only when Dame Kathleen Raven assumed the nurse leadership role in 1958 that any significant impact was achieved with regard to nurses working at ground level.

The reasons for this dramatic shift were obvious. Because of her involvement with the Wood Report, Dame Elizabeth was effectively ostracised by members of her own profession. The AHM in particular launched a sustained and vitriolic campaign in an effort to discredit both Dame Elizabeth and the report. Whereas Dame Elizabeth managed to maintain close contact with the RCN, her influence with regard to other nursing organisations such as the GNC was severely curtailed. Consequently, Dame Elizabeth concentrated on matters largely unrelated to GNC control, for example public health, importation infection control and mental health. The nursing team at Whitehall compiled public health statistics and attempted to switch government focus away from hospital-centred curative healthcare towards preventative community-based healthcare, but this policy initiative met with very little success. The nursing view, however, was endorsed by the World Health Organisation (WHO) which stated that the British system of healthcare delivery 'relied too heavily on the hospital'. The WHO also believed that Britain had the best practical nurses but that they were very poorly educated. The WHO attempted to resolve this problem by drawing Britain's attention to the increasing demand for well-educated nurses, but Britain 'thought itself on top and in no need of education' and failed to respond to WHO concerns.[21] As Dame Elizabeth recalled, individual hospitals were 'far too self-satisfied, they thought they had it all, especially those in London',[22] therefore implementing change was virtually impossible.

If nursing efforts in Whitehall to raise the profile of public health had made little headway, there were at least some encouraging signs in the field of mental health. The NHS had accepted responsibility for psychiatric hospitals and those dealing with the mentally handicapped, although there was an initial reluctance on behalf of the Home Office to supply information relating to these institutions.[23] During the early stages of the NHS, mental health nurses did not form part of the Ministry staff and Dame Elizabeth was instrumental in rectifying this situation. Raising the standards of mental healthcare should, she argued, be a priority. This view was endorsed by members of the CHSC. Subsequently, two psychiatric nurses joined the Ministry team and were responsible for visiting individual mental hospitals in order to obtain relevant information regarding nursing standards. Regional nursing officers were also involved in this process.

Nursing officer reports confirmed the fact that chronic under-staffing in mental hospitals severely affected the quality of patient care, and nursing policy was designed to improve recruitment to the mental health field and upgrade levels of care. The GNC were persuaded to include a period of mental health training in the general nurse syllabus and mental health nurses were encouraged to undertake general nurse training. The interchange of personnel between general and psychiatric nursing sectors was designed to cultivate a wider understanding of mental health work, to raise overall standards of nursing care and, to some extent, to alleviate nursing shortages. However, the Chairman of the CHSC Mental Health Sub-Committee voiced doubts as to the feasibility of this strategy and argued instead for the development of a specialist mental nurse. These doubts were well-founded. Many psychiatric hospitals resisted the introduction of general nurses into their field and only Glasgow gave the scheme wholehearted support.

The 1959 Mental Health Act encouraged a less custodial approach to psychiatric care and mental hospitals became accountable to the Ministry of Health. But despite legislation, outdated procedures and custodial practices in psychiatric care continued. In some instances these practices were shocking. The full extent of physical and emotional abuse suffered by psychiatric patients was not revealed until 1967, with the Ely mental hospital disclosures. Neither could the Ely revelations be viewed in isolation. Evidently, many hospitals were unable to prevent the systematic maltreatment of mental health and mentally handicapped patients. Nurses and ministers were aware of patient abuse from 1950 onwards. The reports received from regional nursing officers regarding mental hospitals were frequently disturbing and ministry officials failed to respond. They believed practices would improve once the mental health field experienced the full impact of NHS changes. Meanwhile regional nursing officers attempted to influence staff in mental hospitals by advocating changes in patient care and by conducting frequent inspections.[24]

Hospitals nonetheless resisted government legislation and new approaches to mental healthcare, and unnecessarily harsh regimes continued to affect inpatient care. However, the overall standard of mental healthcare had improved in many areas by the late 1950s. A nursing course was established which combined the disciplines of public and mental health and a number of hospitals were persuaded to introduce psychiatric treatment on an outpatient basis.[25] Undoubtedly, issues regarding mental health needed to take precedence over general health concerns and a consensus existed to this effect amongst ministers, members of the CHSC and senior nurses, although the nursing commitment at Whitehall to mental health was in part a reflection of Dame Elizabeth's strained relationship with the general nursing sector. The fundamental split that had arisen between the CNO and the nursing establishment over the issue of reform, significantly affected nursing development, primarily because rank and file nurses were reluctant to endorse policy initiatives which emanated from Whitehall.

According to White, nursing influence within government circles declined from 1949 onwards, because the profession had rejected the Wood Report and Bevan's draft proposals for the 1949 Nurses Act. As a result, White argues, Bevan 'felt considerably disillusioned and let down by the nurses' and 'his successors at the Ministry did nothing to further the restructuring of the nursing service'. White further states that nursing issues were treated with 'contempt' by senior civil servants,[26] but no evidence is put forward to support this allegation. More importantly, White makes no distinction between nursing influence at Whitehall during this period and the overall nursing influence within the NHS. Yet this distinction is crucial in order to understand the dynamics of nurse leadership and subsequent professional stagnation. Whereas the NHS reforms had undermined the nursing power base at hospital level, nurses at Whitehall were able to strengthen and expand their spheres of influence, although the CNO between 1948 and 1958 was effectively alienated from the remaining levels of nurse leadership. Dame Elizabeth had assumed the position of CNO intending to initiate and supervise nursing reform; the profession's rejection of reform had forced a shift in priorities. Consequently, while the CNO position exerted considerable political leverage during Dame Elizabeth's term of office, this leverage was not used to strengthen the power base of nurses generally. The NHS had downgraded the role of the matrons and, not surprisingly, Dame Elizabeth had abandoned them to their fate. It was not Bevan and the civil servants who were disillusioned with nurses, but the nurses themselves![27]

The change in leadership in 1958, however, signalled a change in policy direction. Aware of the major gap that existed between Ministry nurses and the nursing establishment,[28] Dame Kathleen Raven, the new CNO, introduced a programme of secondments. Nurse tutors and assistant matrons were invited to spend a period of two years at the Ministry of Health before returning to their normal posts and liaison officers were introduced in order to strengthen links between the Ministry and schools of nursing. The majority of nurses continued to resist change despite these initiatives, both in the area of clinical practice and with regard to professional organisation. Consequently, Dame Kathleen established the Joint Board of Clinical Nursing Studies via the SNAC, to enable the implementation of innovations in nursing practice. In addition, by initiating the Salmon enquiry,[29] the CNO attempted to strengthen the political position of senior nurses at hospital and community level.

Thus, by the 1960s it was possible to detect a shift in the nature of nurse leadership at Whitehall. While Dame Elizabeth had confronted the nursing establishment over the issue of reform, Dame Kathleen chose to bypass resistance and introduce piecemeal reform through a 'back door' route. The leaders had also differed in their approaches to healthcare. Whereas Dame Elizabeth was heavily influenced by the WHO, Dame Kathleen was influenced by the American nursing system. Significantly, following a tour of American hospitals, Dame Kathleen acknowledged that British nurses were completely 'out of date and old-fashioned'.[30] Moreover, American nurses were involved in hospital policy decisions while British matrons were no longer included in any policy formulation, a situation partially rectified by the Salmon reforms. Furthermore, American influence filtered through into nursing practice. The introduction of hospital Intensive Care Units (ICUs) for instance was a prime example of the adoption of American nursing practice. However, although the widespread use of ICUs in Britain became accepted policy, the nursing influence behind this policy has not generally been recognised. As Dame Kathleen recalled, the policy originated with her own report of an American progressive patient care programme. This programme separated patients according to their nursing needs. As a result of a two-month study in Minneapolis and Connecticut, Dame Kathleen compiled an official report 'strongly recommending intensive care units, placing patients needing 24-hour care and life-saving apparatus together in one area of the hospital', since Britain 'could no longer sustain having 15 or 20 patients needing this care scattered in 15 different places over a large hospital'.[31] Having compiled and submitted the report, however, Dame Kathleen was not allowed to sign it - this was 'departmental policy' - but the recommendations were published in medical journals and subsequently implemented as policy. This rather typical scenario explains to some extent why nursing influence has been overlooked and why accounts of nursing history have continually under-estimated the power of nurses at Whitehall.

Clay, for instance, has suggested that in terms of professional structure and healthcare delivery, nurses were 'products of social policy and political forces rather than initiators of policy'.[32] To support this argument, Clay cites the Salmon report of 1966, the Mayston report of 1969 and the Briggs report of 1972,[33] claiming that professional development has been determined by 'external agencies'. However, the Salmon enquiry was initiated by Dame Kathleen and, according to Brian Salmon, the CNO did much of the research work for the Committee. Mayston merely brought community nursing into line with the Salmon recommendations for hospital nursing and the Briggs Committee was established as a result of Dame Kathleen sharing a taxi ride with

Richard Crossman![34] But the invisibility of nurses in the policy-making process has belied their actual level of influence. Policy formulation frequently took place during social gatherings and, since a decision had usually been reached regarding policy directives long before the committee stage, committee meetings were simply a formality. Nurses did not need to dominate committees, therefore, in order to dominate policy. The 'iron triangle' of civil servant, politician and doctor did not pose a major threat to the nursing voice. Doctors may have been outraged by the Salmon proposals to empower nurses, for example, but they were still overruled by politicians and civil servants. The 'iron triangle' could be penetrated and both CNOs stressed their direct contact with the Minister of Health and their ability to effect change.

However, the ability to effect change in nursing policy with regard to patient care and administration should not be confused with the ability to effect changes in the pay and working conditions of nurses, although it is clear that nurses in Whitehall became increasingly involved with the latter issue from 1960 onwards. Dame Elizabeth had experienced little contact with the Treasury, but Dame Kathleen stated that during her term of office regional officers continually advised ministers regarding the pay and conditions of nurses. Moreover, the problem of improving pay and conditions for nurses dominated, and frequently overshadowed, professional development. Furthermore, nurses were attempting to claim professional salaries when they had no criteria for maintaining a professional standard of care. Many of the tasks performed by state registered nurses, state enrolled assistant nurses and ancillary grades were interchangeable. How, then, could state registered nurses justify their claims for increased pay when a person with no training whatsoever was allowed to undertake many of the tasks performed by skilled nurses? A survey conducted by the Confederation of Health Service Employees in support of a Royal Commission into nursing services in 1962 uncovered some alarming facts. The survey, which spanned a total of 206 hospitals, claimed that 'in eighty nine psychiatric hospitals almost 60% of staff were untrained, and in five chest hospitals 74.9% of total staff were untrained'. In addition, the survey stated that in 73 general hospitals there were 'almost two untrained staff for every member of trained staff' and that student nurses were still being left in sole charge of wards, particularly at night. In areas where staff/patient ratios appeared to be reasonable, it was claimed that these favourable ratios were the result of dilution of staff with untrained personnel. Standards of care had fallen and there was an increasing tendency to rely on 'foreign nationals'. One Hampshire hospital, for example, employed '47 foreign nationals out of 145 male nurses, and the students were made up of 3 Latvians, 4 Poles, 2 Austrians, 15 Italians, 4 Spaniards, 2 Chinese, 4 Malayans, 11 Jamaicans and Nigerians'.[35]

The practice of employing foreign nationals, however, was not responsible for the lowering of nursing standards. Professional interest groups had prevented the introduction of training courses for ancillary grade nurses. As nursing practice became more technical in nature, ancillary staff assumed more of the workload previously undertaken by trained staff. By refusing to give adequate instruction to ancillary staff, standards of care were automatically lowered. The nursing profession found itself in a 'catch 22' situation. Improvements in the conditions of service, such as a reduction in working hours, could not be achieved without attracting more recruits; but existing conditions and recruitment practices acted as a deterrent to recruitment. Moreover, the majority of nursing schools were unable to retain student nurses.[36] Therefore, in order to maintain numbers, dilution of trained nurses with untrained personnel was inevitable.

The CNO at the Ministry of Labour, Mrs Bennett, had conducted research into the recruitment and retention problems and acknowledged that the bulk of nursing work was being performed by unskilled workers. However, as Abel-Smith has observed, many patients suffering from chronic disease were nursed entirely by unskilled workers in their own home. Herein lay a crucial problem for qualified nurses. By what criteria did they measure their professional status? The nursing establishment inculcated new recruits with stories of military traditions and the need for a vocational spirit, but this process was no real basis for professional development.

While nurses in Whitehall had managed to penetrate the 'iron triangle' operating from above, they were not able to penetrate the second 'iron triangle' operating from below. Within the nursing establishment, military influence was inextricably linked with religious notions of self-sacrifice and royal patronage.[37] Moreover, it was the military imposition that dominated this triangle of influence. According to Will Hayden, the 'average matron was a sergeant major in a woman's uniform'.[38] Student nurses represented the main body of troops and individual hospitals were administered in much the same way as individual army regiments. Logically, the loyal troops followed matrons' orders; however, these same troops were totally unaware that their commander in chief resided in Whitehall. In contrast to this position, matrons recognised the higher echelons of nurse leadership but chose to ignore their policy initiatives unless they conformed to existing patterns of organisation and practice.[39]

The Nursing Establishment

According to Dame Elizabeth and her colleagues, the nursing establishment consisted of the General Nursing Council, the Royal College of Nursing and the

Association of Hospital Matrons. There were other smaller nursing groups, but these three bodies provided the basis for mainstream nursing opinion. The existence of cross-membership reinforced the 'established' view of professional nursing interests, although one organisation was not necessarily a reflection of another. The GNC and the AHM shared similar anti-educational views regarding nurse training requirements, while at least one section of the RCN recognised the need for an increased educational bias, particularly in relation to post-registration courses. Nevertheless, nursing groups cast doubt on the value of such education and, even where educational support existed, disagreements arose over course outlines and context. Aside from these internal divisions and the rift between Whitehall nurses and the 'establishment', the situation was further complicated by the fact that public health nursing was completely divorced from hospital nursing. The lack of co-operation between ward sisters and public health nurses was described by one senior nurse as 'a kind of subterranean hostility'.[40]

This 'subterranean hostility' reflected the great divide between preventative and curative healthcare, and highlighted a civilian distortion of military healthcare provision. Healthcare within the armed services had concentrated primarily on returning an injured man to the battlefield as quickly as possible, or, if injuries proved too severe for this course of action, discharging him into the civilian community. However, measures were also taken to ensure that the soldier maintained a level of 'bounding good health' and Army medical services provided a 'comprehensive health service to the wives and children of serving soldiers'.[41] Albeit a rather crude comparison, it could be argued that the civilian NHS was far better at 'patching the man up ready for the battlefield' than providing support networks to maintain and promote good health. Vested medical interests also dictated the direction of both military and civilian medicine. Greater emphasis was placed on curative medicine in civilian society, simply because it was considered easier to establish prestige and medical reputation in a curative field than in a preventative one. Subsequently, this emphasis affected the way in which various branches of the nursing profession were viewed. Nurses working within the occupational health field, for instance, were afforded lower status than their counterparts employed in general hospitals. Even within the hospital environment, certain nursing fields lacked prestige. Nurses working with the elderly, chronic sick and mentally ill, for example, were afforded lower status than those working in acute surgical wards and casualty departments. District nurses were considered to be inferior to hospital nurses and the public health sector did not constitute 'real nursing'! However, government investment in public health nursing and the prevention of disease offered a less expensive option in the long term than a continued reliance on curative treatments. As Dr Andrew Topping, Dean of the London School of Hygiene and Tropical Medicine, pointed out:

> ... *the more medical people get to know of the cause of disease, the more those diseases can be avoided. Of the £439 million spent on the NHS, £238 million has gone to the hospitals and a mere 7% of the money went on the prevention of disease.* [42]

Curative treatment continued to take precedence over preventative care and, once the die had been cast in 1948, there appeared to be little room for manoeuvre. As Sir George Godber remarked, from its inauguration onwards the NHS 'could only be deflected in subtle ways over the long term. One could not put a bridle on it and persuade it abruptly to change course'.[43] From a nursing point of view, with the exception of public health nurses and those working in Whitehall, preventative care was a nonentity. Miss E.K. Bally, CNO in Holland County Council, declared that 'it was very difficult to get a nurse with a curative outlook to think in terms of prevention'.[44] It was possible to introduce occasional new courses in public health training, but this was merely tinkering with the system.

While the overall nursing situation reflected this curative versus preventative care scenario, there were also parallels in terms of fixed direction. Once nurses had decided to reject educational reform, they were not likely to deflect from their chosen course. In the character versus intellect debate, character had won the day. The general consensus of nursing opinion had decided that a 'nurse was born not made', practical training therefore ousted theoretical knowledge. However, by 1950 it was clear that views regarding the nursing profession were not entirely restricted to the nursing establishment. During the early years of NHS development it appeared that everyone from dustmen to prison governors held some opinion about nursing. These views which emanated from the general public were varied but did not always merit serious consideration. Many people, for instance, believed that nurses should be allowed to wear make-up because 'attractive nurses cheered up the patients'.[45] Others thought there should be a smarter uniform and a stocking allowance, as was the case with policewomen. Public opinion tended to sway between two extremes: nurses were considered to be prim and efficient, or glamorous and gentle. For recruitment purposes the Ministry of Health had erred on the side of glamour. A photograph of actress Patricia Neale, as she appeared in *The Hasty Heart*, was included in recruitment posters and certain nursing fields were described with glamorous overtones.

There were objections to this 'glamorising' trend. Ipswich Hospital Management Committee, for example, refused to use the Patricia Neale poster, stating that it was up to nurses themselves to decide 'whether they prefer to be represented as glamorous or business-like'.[46] Similarly, a member of Birmingham Regional Hospital Board, Alderman Dingley, was highly critical of a recruitment film entitled *Student Nurse*. The film, he argued, 'over-glamorised surgical nursing in relation to other fields of nursing employment'.[47] But despite objections, the glamour trend continued. Red Cross nurses' uniforms were redesigned by the Queen's dressmaker Norman Hartnell, as were the uniforms of certain prestigious teaching hospitals. Nurses were still digesting the vast army of public opinion when another necessary quality was thrown into the equation. They were informed by the education adviser to the National Association of Girls Clubs, Dr Josephine Brew, that nurses needed to be heroic! Girls and young student nurses required inspiration, she declared: 'the desire to have a hero to worship is so very great'.[48]

According to public opinion, then, nurses were supposed to be prim, efficient, well-disciplined, glamorous, gentle and heroic, and in many respects the nursing profession did conform to this public 'ideal'. There was at least an air of efficiency and nurses were well disciplined. Furthermore, long-standing military participation had supplied nurses with a surfeit of heroines compared to other female professions. They were a bit low in the glamour stakes, but a glut of romantic fiction and television programmes which featured nurses falling in love with every available doctor soon rectified this problem. By conforming to the public ideal, nurses also appeared to gain approval from the medical profession. A study of hospital medical minutes demonstrated a complete lack of demand for educated nurses and some consultants even endorsed the practice of leaving student nurses in charge of wards.[49] This practice was good experience for the girl in training, they argued, and no-one seemed to question whether this same practice was also a good experience for the patients!

However, while nurses were conforming to existing 'ideals', there was no clear definition of the nursing role. As the *Journal of British Nursing* pointed out in 1950:

> *Sometime in the not too distant future, our leaders, if we have any,*
> *will be asked to define nursing and unless they are well prepared*
> *with a clear exposition of the term they will fail.* [50]

Attempts to confront this problem head-on gave rise to intense correspondence between the nursing division at the Ministry of Labour and senior members of the RCN. The nature of this correspondence reveals that nurses themselves were not at all sure of their professional boundaries. Frances Goodall, Secretary to the RCN, sought advice in this matter from the CNO at the Ministry of Labour, Mrs Bennett. The following extract is taken from a letter written by Mrs Bennett dated 2nd May 1951 and sent in reply to Miss Goodall:

> I feel that we should make some attempt at an early date to use a hospital or a ward of a hospital as an experimental centre for giving total patient care; that we should experiment by using different members of the nursing team with other members of the health team, and thus by giving perfect care to a group of people we could find out where the duties of the nurses, almoners, physiotherapists etc. overlap. We could then, I think, sort out the task of the nurse in hospital. [51]

Mrs Bennett continued by proposing possible research subjects, such as:

> ... an examination of the needs of people for nursing care which can be supplied jointly by the public health nursing service and the hospital nursing service. [52]

Other suggestions included the introduction of a period in nurse training which concentrated on community care and connecting nurse training to university education. As Mrs Bennett pointed out:

At the present time the Americans and Canadians consider our training to be useless, or at least poor because we have no university affiliations for basic training. [53]

There was no immediate response to Mrs Bennett's proposals. Frances Goodall had tried to persuade the RCN membership that experimentation was necessary, but to no avail. Nurses generally were resistant to change and believed that existing nursing services were not only adequate but superior to those in Canada and America. Nursing opinion acknowledged that medical equipment and hospital buildings were far better in America and Canada, but they argued that British nursing standards reigned supreme. This view did not reflect international opinion and British Columbia rescinded the long-standing reciprocity agreement with Britain,[54] claiming that nurse education in Britain was substandard. This action forced even the anti-educationalists within nursing to reconsider their stance. Published reviews of an American nursing manual further highlighted the inadequacies of British nurse training. According to the nursing press, the manual contained:

> ... *rather complicated methods of teaching nurses in American schools of nursing. It is based upon psychological studies of learning and is rather difficult to digest. We in England have not yet evolved such specialised methods of teaching our nurses, possibly because we cannot afford to be so leisurely and penetrating.* [55]

Clearly, then, British nurses were not only unable to fully understand the American manual, but were also trying to justify their lack of understanding.

Evidently, British nurses were experiencing a crisis of confidence and some changes in the field of nurse education were needed, if only to restore international prestige. In an attempt to confront this problem, Frances Goodall and educationalists within the RCN launched a fund-raising appeal in order to pay for specialist nurse training courses. However, the wording of the appeal was interesting in that the RCN made an unequivocal statement linking the nursing profession as a whole to military organisation. The appeal, which aimed to raise £500,000, stated that 'after general training the college prepares nurses to be matrons, sisters and nurse administrators in the public health service. These post certificate courses for the officers and NCOs of nursing are dependent on the support of the public'.[56] The appeal was signed by the Countess Mountbatten of Burma and fund raising efforts were conducted in the usual RCN fashion - a series of whist drives, royal garden parties and fetes culminated in a lavish pageant performed at the Royal Festival Hall entitled 'They Carry the Torch'. The cast included 750 nurses and the United Hospitals Choir of 350 voices. The pageant traced the history of nursing and was written as a tribute to the Queen in her coronation year. A replica of Florence Nightingale's lamp was made in Belfast and mounted on Waterloo embankment to shine over the Thames as a symbol of nursing heritage. According to press reports, the pageant was one of the most outstanding musical spectacles ever staged at the Royal Festival Hall, but it also symbolised a fundamental nursing problem - nurses were far more prone to looking backwards into their heroic military history rather than looking forward into the civilian future. Ironically, although some senior nurses had emphasised the need for specialist courses, these were often the same nurses who had vetoed educational reform in terms of basic training. There seemed to be a pervading attitude that only the 'officers' of nursing were entitled to specialist skills. The nursing establishment did not appear to recognise that without fundamental education at basic training level, extra skills could not easily be acquired at 'officer level'.

Although the RCN succeeded in setting up a variety of specialist courses, the content of such courses did not stimulate professional development. Administration courses, for example, were limited and outdated. Within the nursing establishment Frances Goodall had emerged as a leader, but she was unable to gain the full support of the establishment. From the introduction of new courses to persuading nurses to relinquish emoluments in favour of professional salaries, Frances Goodall fought an uphill battle. As the official RCN journal, the *Nursing Times* became increasingly concerned about this lack of policy direction, stating that 'journalistically, to be an official organ is probably a handicap unless the organisation it represents is a pressure group with a clear cut policy'.[57] The RCN was also accused of practising professional apartheid and exerting censorship with regard to nursing articles submitted for publication. Moreover, by the late 1950s RCN membership had dwindled despite the introduction of a generous insurance indemnity for registered nurses. As the *Nursing Times* Advisory Board pointed out, a large number of nurses were displaying a 'curious apathy towards the college'.[58] However, this apathy was predictable rather than curious. Nurses had expected strong leadership from the RCN rather than Frances Goodall operating as a lone voice crying in the wilderness. Although there were RCN members who supported nursing research and education, for at least a decade they were in a minority. Thus, it was not until 1960 that the RCN announced 'the time is ripe for the RCN to give a lead to the profession in the matter of nursing research' and belatedly adopted the principle that 'a profession not rooted in systematic knowledge is a self-contradiction, a myth rather than a reality'.[59]

Professional apartheid also ended in 1960 and, by including registered male nurses, the RCN received an added boost in the drive towards research-based education. From 1960 onwards the RCN moved more confidently in the direction of education. Dingwall *et al* have described this move as a period when nurses began to abandon the Nightingale model of nurse training in favour of the ideas first expounded by Bedford Fenwick.[60] However, it can also be seen as a gradual move away from military influence, particularly as it coincided with the demise of national service. From making statements that had glorified the Empire and endorsed military values, the RCN shifted its stance to embrace intellectual knowledge and, eventually, a degree of radicalism. Thus, in 1954 a series of RCN 'educational lectures' asserted that:

Great Britain has a reputation for maintaining and transmitting the qualities of justice, peace, freedom and integrity, and the nursing profession has a responsibility to see that these qualities continue to be believed in. [61]

In 1960 the rhetoric had changed and the RCN was committed to 'helping nurse leaders of the future to interpret research findings and initiate well devised investigations' into nursing problems.[62] However, the nursing establishment had taken a long time to discover a sense of direction. This was primarily due to a pervading military imposition on nursing development, but the diversity of professional interests within RCN membership did not help the situation. In some respects the nursing establishment had too many leaders, each propounding their individual notions of professionalism but none with an overview of the total problem. Dame Elizabeth had the ability in 1948 to provide this overview, but the CNO was stranded in Whitehall, ostracised by her profession over the issue of reform. Clearly, in terms of professional development, nurses had wasted a decade.

The Outsiders

Aside from the nursing establishment with their concerns of professional legitimacy, there were other, more radical, nursing groups confronting fundamental issues such as hours of work and conditions of service. The largest of these groups (COHSE) sought to improve the pay and conditions of health workers generally. This trade union was less concerned with professional development, and nurse membership was predominantly male. Since female nurses proved reluctant to join trade unions, a separate guild of nurses was constructed within COHSE. This construction was not entirely successful in attracting female recruits; nurses appeared to be conservative not only in outlook but also in political persuasion. As Iris Brook, a founder member, recalled, 'Nurses if they voted at all voted Tory'.[63] Furthermore, standard nurse recruitment practices perpetuated anti-trade union sentiment. Middle-class registered nurses tended to turn their backs on unionism and argued that since nursing was a 'profession not a trade', union membership negated claims for professional status.

This 'professional view' was imposed on student nurses. Some sisters tried to prevent student attendance at union gatherings, and if nurses joined any form of political protest they were victimised as a result. Matrons believed that nurses participating in political action were disgraceful, undignified and unprofessional. In 1948, for instance, a thousand nurses gathered in Hyde Park in London to air their grievances in public. Nevertheless, only one nurse from

London's St Pancras Hospital took part in the demonstration because of the fear of reprisals. Nurse Syms, as the only representative of St Pancras, claimed that although victimisation was indirect, 'anything unprofessional was regarded as serious'.[64] However, with the post-war influx of men into general nursing realms, fear of intimidation lessened. According to Doris Westmacott, a regional COHSE officer during this period, men had a huge impact and influence in general nursing, 'Once male nurses and tutors joined COHSE they encouraged fearful nurses to attend union meetings'.[65]

Despite the significant male impact on the unionisation of general nursing, COHSE nurse membership still consisted primarily of male mental nurses and untrained nursing staff, although state-enrolled assistant nurses (SEANs) also gravitated towards COHSE membership. Many SEANs were part of the larger NHS immigrant workforce and believed that strong union membership was necessary to protect their interests. Immigrant nurses were less concerned about status issues and therefore less inclined to object to the unionisation of nursing generally.

COHSE nurse membership, therefore, differed dramatically from RCN membership and objectives differed accordingly. However, in terms of leadership, COHSE experienced problems. The union was able to reach a consensus regarding general aims and objectives but appeared unable to decide the methods by which objectives could be achieved. The National Executive Council frequently divided into two camps over the issue of overtime bans and other forms of industrial action. Consequently, conference policy decisions were not always implemented. In 1958, for instance, COHSE delegates voted for an overtime ban in selected hospitals, but this policy did not come to fruition. Furthermore, as one of the conference delegates, Mr J. Byrne, stated, this situation did 'reveal a tremendous lack of leadership and facing up to responsibility'. This view was confirmed by another delegate, Mr Chant, in far stronger terms, claiming that, 'In all my years of conference I have never seen such a sorry lack of leadership from the platform. We are not getting anywhere and conference is degenerating into chaos'.[66] Moreover, in many respects the debates surrounding overtime bans proved to be superfluous. The Ministry of Health had pre-empted this move by issuing a directive to hospitals to keep overtime to a minimum and, in some areas, improved recruitment had virtually removed overtime requirements. Therefore, in order to achieve impact, an overtime ban needed to be national in origin rather than selective.

The lack of nurse leadership within COHSE was perhaps more acceptable to nurses than the absence of RCN leadership. As a professional organisation, the

RCN had claimed to represent nursing issues,[67] whereas COHSE was not specifically a nursing union and suffered at times from trying to do all things for all people. Pay disputes[68] usually involved all healthcare workers, and a great deal of union time was spent in attaining professional recognition for a myriad of NHS employees. In terms of pay, for example, the Ministry of Health had refused to recognise theatre technicians' diplomas and there were similar cases of non-recognition throughout the professions allied to medicine. From a nursing standpoint there were several other key weaknesses in union organisation. While the mental nursing sector had achieved some cohesion politically, it was very difficult to challenge the RCN stranglehold on general nursing. More importantly, rank and file nurses were alienated completely from political organisation. In 1963, Frances Goodall of the RCN acknowledged that student and pupil nurses were responsible for undertaking 75% of the nursing work in hospitals, yet these students and pupils had little or no political representation. The RCN included a student nurse association, but this body did not contribute to policy directives and, until 1960, only registered general nurses were able to obtain full membership. COHSE had extended membership to all nursing grades, but matrons had prevented student and pupil nurses from joining unions, although this trend shifted from 1960 onwards as both the RCN and COHSE vied for membership and negotiating strength. Many of the male general nurses had become charge nurses by 1960 and encouraged students and pupils to join unions. The RCN, concerned over falling membership levels, opened its doors to all trained nurses, including men. Furthermore, it can be argued that the RCN was forced to take this action in order to survive since there appeared to be some doubt as to the role of professional bodies within national negotiating frameworks. As the RCN noted in 1966:

> ... if 'protective services', including negotiation of salaries and conditions of service, were to become the prerogative of trade unions, the RCN, as a different organisation, as at present constituted, would inevitably have to retract very considerably. [69]

The relationship between COHSE and the RCN also changed significantly over time. Initially, during the 1950s each organisation attempted to discredit the other and the relationship was one of mutual hostility. The RCN accused COHSE of putting patients at risk by sanctioning strike action and pointed out their distinct lack of nurse leadership, while COHSE attacked the RCN for guarding professional interests and neglecting the conditions of nurses in training. In addition, COHSE also exposed the RCN tendency to relive military nursing traditions and mischievously suggested that the Nightingale legacy had been misinterpreted by the College. The following poem summarised this COHSE view:

> *For years it seems we've heard the tale,*
> *Of dauntless dear Miss Nightingale.*
> *So Royal College please take heed,*
> *And find the leadership you need,*
> *In she who went before.*
> *When ministers her scope would cramp,*
> *She'd set about them with her lamp,*
> *And knock them all for four!*
> *One final point whilst I remember,*
> *She'd be a leading COHSE member.* [70]

Nevertheless, despite the initial antagonistic relationship, a gradual recognition of shared RCN and COHSE objectives had developed by the mid 1960s. In fact, by this stage the nursing establishment generally had accepted the need for some form of political agitation. Subsequently, in 1967, when the GNC was considering a revision of its existing constitution, the Council actually wrote to COHSE asking for suggestions! This move demonstrated a considerable reconciliation between conservative and radical nursing opinion and one which paved the way for greater co-operation from 1969 onwards. Up until this point, however, neither group demonstrated exceptional leadership qualities. The nursing establishment had used military traditions and class boundaries as a precarious foundation for professional status, while COHSE were preoccupied with the interests of all healthcare workers and sometimes failed to give nursing the priority it deserved. The RCN lacked professional direction and COHSE had no national plan to improve the conditions of nurses generally. How did this situation affect the rank and file?

The Rank and File

Throughout the 1950s and 1960s rank and file nurses were working excessively long hours and coping with poor living conditions. As a result, many nurses did not become involved in politics because they were too tired to do so. Others, as previously acknowledged, were prevented from engaging in political activity by over-zealous matrons. Student and pupil nurses tended to believe the rhetoric handed down by previous nursing generations which stated that nursing was an art. Clearly, nurses were required to suffer for this art. Furthermore, many registered nurses believed that students should not actually receive reasonable salaries, as the 'wrong type' of girl would be attracted into the profession.

Nurses needed to dedicate their time to the patients for love rather than money. There appeared to be a prevailing attitude that nurses in training should endure poor conditions and pay as a way of proving their worth and character. Matrons argued that these conditions had been good enough for them and were therefore good enough for the next generation of students. Any moves to reduce working hours and improve nurse pay met with tacit resistance from the Association of Hospital Matrons. During the 1950s, for example, the staff side of the Whitley Council was in the process of negotiating shorter hours; then, only days before an important meeting to discuss policy submissions, the AHM went on record against shorter hours. The AHM decision was based on the traditional Victorian attitude which assumed that nurses should be prepared to work unlimited hours. However, shorter hours for student nurses involved more administrative work for matrons and there is no doubt that this potential increase in workload influenced the AHM stance. While obviously detrimental to students, the matrons' decision not to support shorter hours was also detrimental to patients. Tired nurses made more mistakes and some mistakes were life-threatening. Long hours also hindered recruitment and subsequent understaffing resulted in patient deaths. In one Surrey hospital, for example, a patient broke her leg in an unattended ward and later died. A student nurse had been in total charge of the ward, containing forty patients, and had left it unattended to get herself a drink. A medical spokesman for the hospital admitted that because of severe staffing shortages they were attempting to run wards like communities, with patients doing most of the domestic work.[71]

Although it can be argued that matrons did little to improve the lot of students, the actual expectations of students appeared to be very low. A certain level of acquiescence was maintained by strict discipline and occupational socialisation. Religious notions of self-sacrifice combined with the military concept of duty and obedience to prevent assertiveness and independent thinking. Nurse identification with the military 'officer' class also curbed political participation. Even the feminist tide of the 1970s failed to attract members of the nursing profession. As far as nurses were concerned, women did have authority, the matron was living proof of this fact. Furthermore, while the nursing profession was subordinated to the medical profession in a wider sense, at ground level it was the ward sisters and matrons who exerted control over the students. Nurses lived in fear of the women in authority, not the men! Therefore, nurses generally did not adopt feminist ideology and failed to acknowledge that they were in fact oppressed by both sexes. Nevertheless, male influence in general nursing assisted the unionisation of nursing and, once allowed into the RCN camp, men gave added impetus to the educational wing of the establishment. Therefore, from 1960 onwards, nurses became more politically active. By 1969 the profession had belatedly discovered a sense of direction. In the interim, however, the lack of professional direction and political cohesion had taken its toll on nursing practice.

Nursing Practice

From the Nightingale era onwards, nursing practice was acknowledged to be an art form which demanded skill and dedication. In later years, as a result of nurse participation in the armed services during two world wars, this art of nursing had been subjected to increased levels of regimentation. By 1945 examples of regimentation in nursing practice were numerous. Patients were expected to conform to strict 'tidiness' rules such as having their noses in line with the centre crease of the top bed sheet, keeping their arms by their sides under the bedclothes during matrons' ward inspections, and not cluttering up their bedside lockers with non-essential belongings. Water jugs and glasses were kept in a set order on locker surfaces, as were the vases of flowers. Patients were not allowed to read newspapers in bed because of the risk of print marks on the sheets and visiting hours were adhered to in a rigid fashion. Nurses were expected to ensure that all hospital bed wheels pointed in the same direction, pillowcases placed with the open end away from the door and hospital corners on bed sheets kept at the correct angle. Nursing care was administered with an air of brittle efficiency and task-orientated routines were timed with precision. Student nurses and ancillary workers followed the orders issued by senior staff with blind obedience and an ingrained sense of duty. Moreover, the 20th century concept of military efficiency underpinned existing regimentation and encouraged further military identification in terms of nursing practice.

Nurses and society generally perceived military organisation to be efficient because orders were given and immediately obeyed. Naturally this system provided a level of superficial efficiency; however, no-one actually confronted the fundamental problem of whether or not in the first instance the orders were efficient. Similarly, ward routines appeared to be carried out with efficiency, but no-one questioned the validity of the routines themselves. Furthermore, task-orientated routines were used to reinforce the nursing hierarchy. Whereas, to an extent, the allocation of tasks depended on existing staffing levels, there was no doubt that certain nursing tasks carried more prestige than others. The RCN Horder report[72] had confirmed this hierarchy of nursing skills within nursing practice and had also recommended that 'officer class' nurses should perform the more skilled nursing tasks. Moreover, this recommendation was adopted in theory within professional nursing circles. In practice, staffing levels dictated the allocation of tasks and a nurse's place in the professional hierarchy could change almost on a daily basis. The nursing grade to suffer most from the fluctuations in staffing levels was that of the State Enrolled Assistant Nurse. As Clay has observed:

> ... *at one moment the EN is one of the ward's most lowliest beings, at everyone's beck and call and carrying responsibility without authority; the next, that same nurse is called upon to run the ward because the grade mix has changed and she or he becomes top dog.* [73]

Clearly the SEAN role in the nursing hierarchy was ambiguous and, until 1961, they were forced to call themselves assistants despite their interchangeable roles.

The following poem, written just before SEANs abandoned their prefix of 'assistant', demonstrates the level of ambiguity and resentment experienced by SEANs:

> *Oh staff nurse from your throne so high,*
> *Look down with pity on such as I.*
> *In three short years you're at the top,*
> *While I'm still busy with the mop.*
> *For after years of hardest labour,*
> *I'm still not fit to be your neighbour.*
> *I walk behind you through the door,*
> *A bottle spilt I clean the floor.*
> *The staff nurse gently milks my brains,*
> *But I'm still sluicing at the drains.*
> *'How does one lay up for a lumbar puncture?'*
> *Then 'empty bottles at this juncture'.*
> *I may not even raise a frown,*
> *At enemas given upside down.*
> *I humbly thank you for your blessings,*
> *While cleaning away your dirty dressings.*
> *To be left in charge is quite unheard,*
> *Any first year nurse may give us the bird.*
> *Alas too late one learns the folly,*
> *One gets the work but not the lolly.*
> *From June the 30th I remain persistent,*
> *State Enrolled Nurse please - not ASSISTANT.* [74]

Enrolled nurses were exploited on a regular basis, but they were at least trained. Therefore, when required to take responsibility for a ward, most were able to rise to the occasion. The same could not be said for student nurses, who were exploited in much the same way as enrolled nurses. A survey undertaken by the Nuffield Hospitals Trust in 1953 revealed that many student nurses were left in charge of wards for at least one-fifth of their working hours. As the survey report stated:

> ... this state of affairs was a source of apprehension to many nurses because their experience to date was inadequate to enable them to meet the demands which might be made on them. [75]

In theory, ward sisters were supposed to instruct student nurses within the practical setting and to prepare them for positions of responsibility, but in practice they had little time to conduct formal teaching sessions. The Nuffield survey claimed that over a weekly period the highest figure recorded for teaching purposes was 11 hours and the lowest figure 7 minutes. Some ward sisters maintained that formal teaching was not necessary; they believed that students were taught in the normal course of the day, simply by working alongside trained staff and by picking up information as they worked. The Nuffield survey discovered that only one sister spent more than 25% of her time directly associating with students, the remainder spent between 5% and 19% of their time with students. Much of this time was dedicated to the giving and receiving of reports and instruction in nursing techniques was negligible. In some instances the medical conditions of patients were not explained to students, and sisters assumed that information would somehow 'filter through'.

Staff nurses appeared, on average, to spend more time working alongside students, but this time was usually dedicated to 'basic nursing care' such as pressure point rounds and bed-making. The repetitive nature of these tasks provided little opportunity for teaching. Student nurses administered nursing care within a regimental routine and frequently had no idea why certain tasks were being performed, or the significance of medical changes in a patient's condition. It was not surprising, therefore, that students were apprehensive when left in charge of wards. Furthermore, the lack of ward teaching became increasingly dangerous as medical technology forced nurses to shift away from their 'art' and embrace the ideas of science.

Regimented nursing routines were, nonetheless, challenged by new ideas of nursing care. For instance, the concept of nursing by 'case assignments', whereby different levels of nurse seniority merged and basic nursing was shared on an equal basis. (The normal ward routine is demonstrated in Table 6.1 and example patterns of student nurse work are outlined in Tables 6.2, 6.3 and 6.4.)

Table 6.1
The daily routine of a ward (based on the practice of the majority of the wards observed)

Hours	Basic Nursing	Technical Nursing	Ward Organisation	Domestic	External Contacts[a]
0000-0100	..	..	..	..	3
0100-0200	..	Stockmaking	Reports	..	3
0200-0300	..	Medical investigations[b]	..	..	..
0300-0400	..	Medical investigations	..	..	3
0400-0500	Washing round	Medical investigations	..	..	..
0500-0600	Morning tea; bed-making; pressure areas; bedpans and urinals	Injections; medical investigations	..	..	..
0600-0700	Bedpans and urinals; bed-tidying	TPRs; injections; medical investigations	..	Sweep main ward floor; clean office	..
0700-0800	Breakfasts	Medicines; sterilisation; medical investigations	Reports; charting		..
0800-0900	Bed-tidying; pressure areas; bedpans and urinals; water glass round	Sputum mugs; medical investigations	Stores; charting; flowers	Sort soiled linen; dust, tidy ward; polish ward floor; scrub ancillary rooms	1, 2, 3
0900-1000	Bed-tidying; pressure areas; water glass round	Medicines; injections; dressings; sputum mugs sterilisation	Stores; charting; flowers		
1000-1100	Elevenses; water glass round	Injections; dressings; sterilisation	Stores; charting	Sort soiled linen; dust, tidy ward; scrub ancillary rooms	1, 2
1100-1200	Water glass round	Dressings; stockmaking; sterililsation	Stores; charting	Sort soiled linen; scrub ancillary rooms	1, 2
1200-1300	Dinners	Stockmaking	..	..	3
1300-1400	Bed-tidying; bed-bathing; pressure areas; washing round; bedpans and urinals	Medicines; injections; stocktaking	..	Sort clean linen	2, 3
1400-1500	Bed-making; washing round; bed-bathing	Stockmaking	..	Sort clean linen; locker round	1, 2, 3, 4
1500-1600	Bed-making; bed-bathing	Stockmaking	..	Sort clean and soiled linen; tidy kitchen	1, 2, 4
1600-1700	Teas; bedpans and urinals; bed-making; bed-bathing	TPRs	Charting	Sort clean and soiled linen; tidy kitchen	2, 3
1700-1800	Bed-making; bed-bathing; bed-tidying	Medicines; injections	Charting	Sort clean and soiled linen; sweep ward floor	1
1800-1900	Suppers; pressure areas	Injections; sputum mugs	Charting	Sort soiled linen	..
1900-2000	..	Dressings; stockmaking	Reports; charting; flowers	Sort soiled linen	3, 4
2000-2100	Night drinks; bed-tidying; bedpans and urinals; pressure areas	Sterilisation	Flowers	Sort soiled linen	..
2100-2200	..	Medicines; injections	..	..	..
2200-2300	..	..	..	..	..
2300-2400	..	..	..	..	..

Notes:
[a] 1 = medical staff; 2 = external departments (for X-ray, blood speciment, basal metabolic rate, electrocardiograph)
3 = nurses' meal breaks; 4 = visitors.
[b] E.g. gastric contents tests.

Source: The Nuffield Hospital Trust Survey 1953

Table 6.2
Examples of pattern of work of individual first-year nurses

Task	Hours spent in one week by nurse							
	A	B	C	D	E	F	G	H
Management								
Instructions	—	1.7	—	—	—	—	3.1	—
Tuition	—	—	—	—	—	—	*1.2*	—
Out of ward on official duties	—	1.5	—	1.0	—	—	2.6	—
Technical nursing								
Dressings	2.3	2.4	—	—	—	—	—	2.1
Medicines	*1.9*	*1.4*	—	—	—	—	—	*1.0*
Preparation of procedures	1.9	5.1	—	—	—	—	—	1.4
Temperature, pulse, respiration	*2.8*	—	—	—	*2.7*	*1.2*	—	—
Nursing procedures	—	2.2	—	—	..	—	—	1.4
Urine measurements	—	—	—	*1.7*	—	—	—	—
Basic nursing								
Bedmaking	7.1	3.8	—	7.6	6.0	4.8	1.5	3.4
Bed tidying	*2.8*	—	—	—	*1.9*	*5.1*	*1.0*	—
Food to patients	6.4	—	15.3	12.2	8.1	7.0	8.7	15.0
Blanket bathing	—	—	—	*1.9*	—	*2.9*	—	*1.3*
Toilet rounds	—	2.1	—	1.7	—	—	—	—
Bedpans	*7.2*	—	*11.6*	*4.2*	*6.9*	*4.7*	—	*3.6*
Care of pressure areas	4.9	—	—	2.1	—	1.1	1.5	2.2
Screens	*1.7*	—	*1.8*	*1.2*	*1.9*	—	—	*1.0*
Assistance to patients	—	2.1	—	—	1.0	—	—	1.0
Personal contact with patients	—	—	—	—	*1.0*	*1.3*	*2.2*	—
Feeding patients	—	—	—	—	—	—	2.2	1.3
Water glass round	—	*1.7*	—	—	—	—	—	—
Sluicing	—	—	—	1.0	—	—	1.3	—
Admissions	—	—	—	—	—	*1.0*	—	*1.1*
Domestic								
Light cleaning	4.0	4.3	6.4	4.3	6.1	4.2	5.7	—
Heavy cleaning	—	—	*2.7*	—	—	—	*1.5*	—
Total hours spent on main tasks	43.0	33.2	37.8	38.9	35.6	33.3	32.5	35.8
Hours spent on tasks each occupying less than 2% of working time	5.0	14.8	10.2	9.1	12.4	14.7	15.5	12.2

Source: The Nuffield Hospital Trust Survey 1953

Table 6.3
Examples of pattern of work of individual second-year nurses

Task	Hours spent in one week by nurse			
	A [a]	B	C [b]	D
Management				
Instructions	1.7	1.5	2.9	1.2
Clerical work	—	—	*1.4*	—
Out of ward on official duties	2.6	—	—	2.1
Technical nursing				
Dressings	2.6	1.5	—	4.4
Medicines	—	*2.1*	—	*1.4*
Preparation of procedures	3.2	3.6	1.4	4.9
Temperature, pulse, respiration	*2.0*	*3.0*	*1.7*	—
Stockmaking	1.4	—	—	1.5
Basic nursing				
Bedmaking	4.7	4.5	2.1	4.0
Bed tidying	*2.0*	*1.5*	*1.6*	*2.8*
Food to patients	4.5	3.9	7.1	7.7
Blanket bathing	*1.1*	—	*1.2*	*1.1*
Toilet rounds	—	—	1.3	—
Care of pressure areas	*2.1*	*4.9*	*1.8*	—
Bedpans	1.7	—	—	—
Screens	—	*1.6*	—	—
Personal contact with patients	1.9	1.3	2.5	2.2
Domestic				
Light cleaning	3.3	2.8	2.2	1.3
Total hours spent on main tasks	34.8	32.2	27.2	34.6
Hours spent on tasks each occupying less than 2% of working time	13.2	15.8	20.8	13.4

Notes:

[a] Worked in modified case assignment ward.

[b] Acting staff nurse

Source: The Nuffield Hospital Trust Survey 1953

Table 6.4
Examples of pattern of work of individual third-year nurses

Task	Hours spent in one week by nurse					
	A[a]	B[b]	C	D	E	F
Management						
Reports	—	3.9	—	—	—	2.5
Instructions	*2.7*	*3.2*	*1.3*	*1.4*	*3.0*	—
Clerical work	1.3	1.1	—	—	1.4	—
Charting work	*1.2*	—	—	—	—	*2.5*
Out of ward on official duties	—	1.2	3.2	5.5	—	—
Technical nursing						
Time spend with doctors	—	2.6	—	—	1.0	2.0
Dressings	—	*9.8*	*5.1*	*1.4*	—	—
Medicines	2.2	—	—	2.4	4.8	7.2
Nursing procedures	*1.5*	*2.3*	*1.1*	—	*1.5*	*2.3*
Preparation of procedures	1.5	3.9	2.4	2.3	2.7	1.6
Temperature, pulse, respiration	*1.4*	—	—	*3.5*	*1.0*	—
Urine testing	—	—	1.1	—	—	—
Stockmaking	—	*2.0*	—	—	—	—
Basic nursing						
Bedmaking	2.8	2.5	2.4	5.6	7.8	4.3
Bed tidying	—	—	*1.1*	—	*1.2*	*1.2*
Food to patients	5.6	—	5.2	5.9	5.0	3.7
Blanket bathing	*1.3*	—	—	—	*1.6*	—
Toilet rounds	—	—	1.8	1.1	—	2.1
Care of pressure areas	—	—	*1.2*	—	—	*2.4*
Bedpans	—	—	—	1.6	1.0	—
Personal contact with patients	*2.2*	*1.5*	—	*1.2*	*1.5*	*1.6*
Domestic						
Light cleaning	2.1	—	—	—	—	—
Total hours spent on main tasks	**27.2**	**34.0**	**25.9**	**31.9**	**33.5**	**33.4**
Hours spent on tasks each occupying less than 2% of working time	20.8	14.0	22.1	16.1	14.5	14.6

Notes:

[a] Worked in modified case assignment ward.

[b] Acting staff nurse

Source: The Nuffield Hospital Trust Survey 1953

But these challenges were offset by certain medical procedures that demanded regimentation, particularly in relation to time discipline. Thus there were conflicting arguments for and against regimentation.

Regimentation in Nursing Practice

The degree of regimentation in nursing practice varied between hospitals, and sometimes even between wards of hospitals. Ward sisters with military experience were more likely to adhere to authoritarian regimes, for instance, than sisters who had trained and remained in the civilian field. Moreover, hospitals situated near naval, army and air force bases tended to employ more ex-service personnel and were therefore more 'military' in style and atmosphere than hospitals situated elsewhere. In many respects, however, the distinctions between civilian and military nursing practices were completely blurred. Evidently, most disagreements regarding nursing techniques at ward level occurred not between military and civilian nurses but between 'old school' and 'new school' military nurses. Joan Markham, an ex-naval nurse, described the transition from service to civilian nursing after 1945 as a period which provoked a 'clash' on the wards. Second World War military nurses were accustomed to the early ambulation of patients, for example, whereas civilian sisters, even those with earlier military experience, were convinced that early ambulation would prove to be life-threatening. Some sisters even argued that early ambulation should be discouraged on the grounds that the process interfered with ward tidiness.[76] Similarly, nurses with recent military experience had administered penicillin to patients and recognised that practices such as the application of poultices to wounds were rendered superfluous by this drug. Yet within the civilian field nurses insisted that these outdated techniques were of value. This ludicrous situation provided the most valid argument for nursing research. The value of nursing procedures needed to be proved, rather than to be performed out of habit.

However, nursing routines did more than reinforce the hierarchy and perpetuate outmoded practice. Organising work as a series of routines provided an important emotional barrier between the nurse and patient. Case assignment care, whereby a nurse was assigned a number of patients and administered their total care, threatened this barrier.[77] Therefore, case assignment nursing methods were not popular in many quarters, despite the fact that in terms of time management it was more practical to redress a patient's wound at the same time as performing a blanket bath. Similarly, any patient observations such as temperature recordings could be taken at the same time. Undoubtedly patients would benefit from this total care scenario in that most nursing procedures would be confined to a limited period, enabling the patient to relax for the remainder of the time. Nevertheless, the fact that one nurse was required to spend far more time than usual with individual patients proved to be a major stumbling block for case assignment nursing, not only because the system eroded barriers in nurse/patient relationships, but also because poor staffing levels precluded the monopolisation of one nurse by one patient for any length of time.

Nurse routines also provided an 'air of efficiency', although a brief examination of ward organisation in Table 6.1 demonstrates that, in practice, most routines were actually highly inefficient. Even without adopting case assignment nursing, adjustments could have been made at a basic level to increase efficiency. For instance, there was no reason why a patient's sputum mug could not be changed while the patient was receiving a blanket bath rather than justifying a 'sputum round'. Patient observations such as temperature, pulse and respiration rate were recorded at least twice a day, and in some wards on a four-hourly basis as a matter of course. These frequent observations were only necessary for a minority of patients, most required only daily observation recordings. There were some sisters who also insisted on recording daily urinalysis for all patients, regardless of their medical condition.

Even necessary nursing procedures could be described as inefficient, as the Nuffield survey pointed out:

> *Ingenuity and common sense could achieve a great deal. The placing of equipment in the ward does not always seem to be related to convenience of use. Thus, in order to fill a hot water bottle the nurse has been observed to fetch it from one room, take it to another to fill it, procure a cover from yet another and finally carry it to the patient in the ward. It is not, in fact, surprising to find that a nurse may walk 2 miles a day in the course of her work. Nurses themselves could cut out some of this without incurring any alterations to the ward and its equipment. Though 194 hours during a 26-week period were taken up with moving the screens around patients' beds. In some wards these screens had no wheels and required considerable effort to move them from place to place. If screens were replaced by curtains around patient beds, time and effort would be saved.* [78]

The Nuffield survey concluded that nurses made work for themselves and that outdated routines remained the biggest obstacle to overall efficiency. The survey cited many examples of inefficiency in nursing practice and argued that nursing attitudes needed to change. As the report stated, 'once it is accepted by nurses that to plan to save time and unnecessary effort is wholly desirable, the chief obstacle to improvement on these lines will have been overcome'.[79] Rigid routines and procedures, however, were popular with nurses, not least because they provided security. For example, if nursing procedures were followed to the letter and a patient's condition deteriorated regardless, a nurse could be exonerated from any blame. In this way nurses were protected by the rigidity of nursing practice. As Maclean has noted:

> *In places where precision is essential and time is at a premium, a military style operation has obvious advantages. There is simply no room for individual error and the medical and senior nursing personnel rightly expect prompt, standardised responses to demands.* [80]

The need for standardised responses to medical emergencies, however, did not excuse the ongoing lack of flexibility in nursing practice; although this lack of flexibility was partly due to professional insecurity since, in the absence of appropriate theoretical education, nursing responsibilities were disproportionate to the nursing knowledge base.

Nurses, nonetheless, did not exclusively control the administration of patient care, and changes in medical practice exerted conflicting influences on task-orientated routines. The increasing amount of patient contact with departments outside the ward environment interrupted basic routines. Similarly, frequent visits to the ward by specialist personnel such as physiotherapists, occupational therapists, laboratory technicians and radiographers caused considerable disruption. Even the long-established ward round conducted by medical consultants became subjected to 'outside influences'. Ward rounds were delayed if a patient's X-rays or blood sample results were unavailable at a given time, for instance, or if a patient was away from the ward receiving treatment in a specialist department. Consequently, because it was impossible to predict medical and specialist ward visits with any degree of certainty, ward sisters were increasingly unable to plan their working day. Therefore, nurses ploughed through the day adhering to routines that were subjected to constant interruption. More importantly, some patients missed out on aspects of nursing care as a result of this process. If patients were in the X-ray department while pressure points were being attended to, for example, they were often excluded from pressure area care altogether because the round had been missed. Nurses were sometimes able to remember which patients had missed certain treatments, but whether or not these treatments were performed later in the day depended on staffing levels and the time schedule of remaining routines.

Conversely, some medical procedures and increased specialism reinforced regimentation in nursing practice. Advances in drug therapy, the administration of intravenous infusions, blood transfusions and new surgical techniques, all combined to dictate methods of patient care. Many of the medical diagnostic procedures were potentially life-threatening and the increased risks to patients undergoing treatment resulted in the implementation of new guidelines which governed the observation of such patients. These new regulations relied heavily on systematic routines to ensure accurate recordings of a patient's condition. Scientific medicine, therefore, introduced science-related disciplines. There was also a danger noted by Titmuss that the 'discipline, required by science for the practice of medicine, could become an end in itself'.[81] However, it was not merely medical technology that increased the reliance on ward routines. In some instances, medical ideas were enough to reinforce regimentation. For example, Guttman's work with paraplegic patients from 1945 onwards was aimed at improving the quality of life for such patients. Guttman's ideas relied on a strict nursing regime that involved turning patients on a two-hourly basis in order to prevent pressure sores and expressing patients' bladders four-hourly to prevent urinary infections. Such was Guttman's commitment to this regime that he regularly descended on wards in the middle of the night to check that nurses were carrying out his orders.[82] Task orientation, therefore, was not only popular with nurses but frequently endorsed by members of the medical profession. Moreover, it was not until the early 1960s that some nurses began to question the value of routines and simultaneously challenge the foundations of nursing.

Art versus Science

In many respects, the art versus science debate within nursing reflected the character versus intellect debate. These debates in turn were connected to the wider issue of care versus cure in nursing and medical practice. Nurse leaders within the RCN and GNC had not clearly defined the nursing role and many regarded nursing as being purely vocational rather than professional in nature. In an attempt to define occupational interests, the *Journal of British Nursing* dedicated an editorial to 'The Beauty that is Nursing', describing the glory and 'incorruptible rewards' which could be gained from nursing, and the editorial adopted a patronising attitude towards lesser professions! The *Journal of British Nursing* did not represent all nursing opinion, but it was clear that many nurses did believe in occupying the moral high ground with regard to other professions. The editorial merely reflected this nursing stance, as the following extract demonstrates:

> *In these times of collective bargaining, when groups of individuals bound together in identical trades and professions, meet for the purpose of bettering their living conditions, shortening their hours of work and demanding increased weekly wages, one is neither surprised nor yet critical of their actions. Their work is not sufficiently enthralling, nor so vital to the community as is nursing. Not for them is the glory and satisfaction of helping to wrest a sick child from the jaws of death, nor to bind up broken and bleeding limbs, nor to soothe the pain of others in their weakness. They must earn money to buy their satisfaction and feeling of wellbeing. Ours is in our daily work.* [83]

The moral tone and emotional content of this editorial amounted to little more than self-glorification. The assumption that nurses should consider themselves well blessed compared to other occupations was no more than a value judgement. More importantly, judgements of this kind did not clarify the nursing role. This in itself was not surprising; nurses themselves appeared unaware of their roles, except perhaps in the very broad sense of contributing to the relief of suffering. However, one of the typical educationalists within the RCN, Norah Mackenzie, enumerated the exact duties of the nurse as follows:

1. *The intelligent relief of suffering.*
2. *The restoration of health.*
3. *Maintenance of health.*
4. *The provision of a stable group, i.e. the nursing profession.*
5. *The transmission and handing on of the craft of nursing.*
6. *The production of individual democratic citizens.*
7. *The maintenance of the values of justice, peace, freedom and integrity.* [84]

The rhetoric which emanated from a series of lectures given by Norah Mackenzie failed to explain how these duties were to be performed in the long term and, given the lack of nurse education, how 'intelligent relief of suffering' could be accomplished. Instead, the lectures concentrated on how certain desirable values should be upheld and how nurses needed to adopt a good posture and a pleasing voice to reassure their patients. As Mackenzie asserted, 'We have three years to teach the students how to speak and move with easy and serene gestures'[85] and clearly science did not have a part to play in this form of training!

In fact, science was barely mentioned in RCN nursing lectures, except to acknowledge that some nurses arrived in the preliminary training school with a good science background. There appeared to be a general distrust of science, not in terms of immunisation programmes and drug therapy but in terms of nursing practice. Nurses were reluctant to attend to a patient's psychological needs, for instance, fearing that this change in focus would detract from nursing as a craft. Furthermore, while nurses in Whitehall had been encouraging greater co-operation between community and hospital nursing services, nursing lectures frequently stressed the supremacy of hospital nurses. Mackenzie even argued that it was a 'pity' that the flow from hospital to occupational health work could not be stemmed, and stated that 'I would like to feel that the life in the hospital and on the wards gave such satisfaction that the qualified did not wish to leave it'.[86] The problem of precisely who was supposed to nurse in the community and industrial fields, if qualified nurses failed to leave the hospital environment, was not confronted, neither was the problem of ignorance with regard to science.

There were many situations where nurses rejected science and research, and nursing approaches to fundamental care provided the clearest example. A wide variety of pressure sore treatments existed, for instance, which did not vary according to the severity of pressure sore risks encountered by patients, but depended on the personal preference of individual ward sisters. Once pressure sores had developed they were treated with applications of honey on some wards and egg white and oxygen on others. More painfully, many sisters treated sores with applications of iodine in the belief that a patient's skin would be toughened in the process. The work undertaken by Guttman had proved that pressure sores were prevented by constantly relieving pressure but this information was only slowly absorbed by the nursing profession.

Patients were also subjected to saline baths as, during the war, it had been noted that wounded servicemen who were abandoned in the sea for any length of time experienced an acceleration in the healing process, until nurses eventually realised that the quantity of salt normally added to a patient's bath did not achieve the same effect as sea water.[87] Similarly, the application of wound poultices and the administration of inhalations continued despite the widespread use of antibiotics. The need for nursing research was clearly apparent. Studies of patient care using scientific guidelines could potentially predict reactions to various nursing treatments, and standards of nursing could be measured and evaluated. While the art of nursing was gradually being replaced by various scientific developments, the medical profession also experienced a similar shift. As Titmuss observed, old empiricisms in medicine had assumed the proportions of an authoritarian art, whereas new techniques enabled the 'merest houseman to confound a consultant's argument with a little sheet of paper from the laboratory'.[88] As medicine became more beholden to science, the nursing position was equally usurped by a multiplicity of other healthcare professionals.

Professional Boundaries

The erosion of the 'art' base in nursing practice, and the lack of professional direction, placed nurses in an occupational limbo land. At one extreme the nurse was a technician, capable of taking intravenous blood samples, while at the other she was a domestic, cleaning out the sluice and disinfecting ward equipment. Between these two extremes nurses assumed their responsibilities according to the skill mix of available staff and the demands placed upon them by patients and medical personnel. At times, therefore, a nurse's work impinged on the work of a doctor and frequently overlapped with work undertaken by other healthcare professionals.

This lack of clearly defined professional boundaries involved considerable risks for nurses. They could, for instance, be accused of negligence should patients suffer as a result of certain procedures, regardless of whether the procedures were performed correctly. Indemnity insurance afforded to nurses was negligible compared to that of the medical profession, yet it was often nurses rather than doctors who assumed the blame for medical errors. The vulnerability of nursing practice in relation to medical practice was exposed in 1949 when a patient died from receiving the wrong injection during a minor operation. A student nurse had drawn up the injection from the wrong bottle and a doctor had administered the drug without checking the bottle label. According to the coroner, no blame could be attached to the hospital, dispensary or doctor for this mistake; it was concluded that the patient had died as a result of nurse incompetence. More importantly, the coroner stated that 'a doctor must be able to rely on a competent nurse that the material he is injecting is the right one. It is quite fantastic to suggest that he approach every solution with suspicion'.[89]

However, it can be argued that it was really 'fantastic' to suggest that doctors should treat nurses, student or trained, as though they were infallible. But nurses continued to bear the brunt of responsibility in situations where they assisted medical practice and increasingly became scapegoats for medical errors. Nurses were also at risk when carrying out technical nursing procedures and their vulnerability stifled professional development. Since the RCN provided legal support for registered nurses, this body was understandably cautious when sanctioning new nursing procedures. The RCN offered indemnity insurance to nurses, but did not wish to be involved in constant legal battles as this would inevitably drain limited financial resources.

In order to protect the nursing position, a system of drug checking evolved which excluded the doctor. Two nurses were held responsible for ascertaining the accuracy of drug administration and were required to sign appropriate prescription sheets. Nurses were also advised by the RCN to refrain from performing medical tasks. This advice posed a problem for many nurses. There appeared to be a wide variation between individual hospitals regarding the functions of a nurse, and tasks which were interpreted as nursing in one hospital were considered to be medical in another. These interpretations also changed over a period of time. In the 1950s, for example, distinctions between medical and nursing tasks were blurred in the areas of catheterisation, the taking of blood pressure, urine testing and the taking of blood specimens, whereas in the 1960s the dividing line had shifted and debates regarding the overlap of medical and nursing practice centred on whether nurses should be allowed to perform electrocardiographs and administer intravenous drugs. Throughout these debates the RCN issued constant warnings since, if nurses entered what the RCN considered to be a medical arena, they would increase their liability risk in nursing practice. In view of these warnings the nurse as technician was slow to evolve.[90]

Legal concerns prevented nurses from establishing a technical role, but there were no such barriers at the other end of the scale. Nurses performed a myriad of domestic tasks: washing up, dusting, polishing, sluicing linen and cleaning toilets, to name but a few. However, many ward orderlies carried out nursing tasks such as giving out hot water bottles, feeding patients and sterilising crockery. A dividing line between domestic and nursing duties simply did not exist in most hospitals. The workload was allocated according to staff availability rather than to spheres of influence and relative skills, although the way in which tasks were allocated also depended on the position of staff within the overall nursing hierarchy. Thus, two staff members of a similar status would be graded according to the length of time employed at the hospital. Even with regard to ward orderlies, the person employed for the longest period assumed seniority and, therefore, performed less distasteful tasks than her subordinates.

Nurses strictly adhered to the principle of 'time' seniority. This principle posed particular problems when nurses were required to relieve staff on wards other than their own. When a registered nurse was sent as additional help to another ward, the first question she was asked was 'when did you qualify?' If the qualifying date of the relief nurse preceded that of the established nurse, then the latter relinquished her authority. Consequently, relief nurses could assume control of specialised wards without appropriate nursing experience. The practice of 'time' seniority therefore was dangerous in that it involved considerable risks to patients. The practice was also inefficient since relief nurses did not always know where various equipment was stored, and a considerable amount of time was wasted in ascertaining the ward layout.

The concept of 'time seniority' in civilian nursing practice was a direct military legacy. Except for the most senior posts in the military, which were filled on the basis of careful selection procedures, all promotions were conducted on the basis of 'time served'. Within the military nursing services, registered nurses were frequently required to act as relief nurses in a variety of specialties. However, the relief system that worked in military circles was unworkable in the civilian nursing sector because of fundamental differences in training. Since wartime conditions demanded flexibility, registered nurses in the armed forces did not remain in one post for longer than two years. Military medical requirements dictated that, in some respects, nurses were 'Jack of all trades and master of none'.[91] This flexibility rule ensured that military relief nurses were experienced in most specialties, while in the civilian nursing field it was not uncommon for registered nurses to remain in the same specialty for their entire career. Civilian nurses were not therefore equipped to operate an efficient relief system. This tendency of civilian nurses to remain in one post for a considerable length of time also contributed to professional stagnation and a cloistering of ideas. Military nursing services did not experience the same staffing problems as the civilian sector, and differences in staffing levels alone allowed for greater flexibility in nursing practice.[92]

Recruitment figures for the military nursing services remained high until the late 1960s when, according to military personnel, figures dropped as a result of the media coverage given to the Vietnam War. By the late 1960s military nurses had endorsed professionalism, combined specialism with flexibility and embraced the concept of teamwork. Meanwhile, their civilian counterparts were struggling to maintain a hierarchy of skills in nursing practice, encumbered by an outdated military model of nursing organisation.

Conclusion

It was clear that nurses failed to take control of professional direction in the early stages of National Health Service development. For at least a decade, national nurse leaders able to influence policy decisions were effectively ostracised from 'mainstream' nursing opinion. White has argued that 'during the years 1948-1961 the central reference for decisions rested on a search for status',[93] but nurses were clearly not searching for a new status. Instead, they were employing every means at their disposal to maintain an old one, which relied heavily on military identification. Nurse leaders were unable to penetrate the formidable 'iron triangle' of military influence, royal patronage and religious beliefs that dominated the policies of the nursing establishment. It was only when the military ethos within society as a whole began to subside with the demise of National Service that a corresponding shift away from military identification could be detected within nursing circles. This shift gathered momentum because advances in medical science forced a move towards research-based rather than task-orientated nursing practice.

The 1953 Nuffield survey and subsequent reports had observed that skilled nurses were not to be found working at the patient's bedside. As nurses progressed within the hierarchy of nursing practice, they became more involved with administration. In theory, registered nurses were trained for administrative tasks and the enrolled nurse for bedside care, but in practice the roles were interchangeable. The introduction of a clinical career structure for the enrolled nurse may have resolved this problem. Nurse recruitment may also have benefited from this move since many girls were reluctant to embark on enrolled nurse training because of the lack of career opportunities. But a system which allowed for a parallel promotional structure alongside registered nurses was not even considered, let alone implemented. The enrolled nurse was forced to take her place in the nursing hierarchy beneath the registered nurse.

Debates regarding nursing practice failed to reach a satisfactory compromise since there was no recognition that a nurse's character could benefit from intellectual knowledge, or that scientific techniques could be used to underpin the 'art' of nursing. Nurses also failed to acknowledge that, although medical science demanded some level of regimentation, total reliance on routines merely reinforced the nursing hierarchy and reduced efficiency levels. There were no professional boundaries vis-a-vis other healthcare workers and fundamental problems associated with nursing development reflected much wider difficulties of professional alignment.

Endnotes

(1)   White, *op. cit.*
(2)   S. Haywood and D.J. Hunter, 'Consultative processes in health policy in the United Kingdom: a view from the centre', *Policy Administration*, 69 (1982), p.152-4
(3)   Hart *op. cit.*, p.176
(4)   U. Maclean, *Nursing in Contemporary Society* (1974), p.108
(5)   M. Broadley, *Patients are People* (1995), p.87
(6)   The mental health field was less affected by changes in medical technology although advances in drug therapy enabled more patients to be treated on an outpatient basis. However, once the responsibility for training psychiatric nurses was transferred to the GNC, the mental health field embarked on a period of regimentation as the GNC struggled to make mental nursing techniques and routines conform to those of general nursing.
(7)   Titmuss, *op. cit.*, p.201
(8)   Issues of professional alignment in a wider sense are addressed in Chapter 6.
(9)   A comparison between military and civilian nurses from 1945 onwards reveals that military nurses fared much better in terms of professional development since military nurses were forced to follow their leadership. Military nurses also achieved a greater level of political influence within the services because they were competing on the same terms as men, i.e. women were single, without children and enjoyed the back-up of domestic support.
(10)   *Daily Graphic*, 2nd July 1948; part of a collection of press cuttings held at the RCNA (RCN/4/39) which also includes extracts from the *British Medical Journal, The Times, Sunday Mercury, Evening Chronicle* and the *Nursing Times.*
(11)   RCNA RCN/4/39. *British Medical Journal*, 26th June 1948
(12)   White, *op cit.*, p.272
(13)   Splane and Splane, *op. cit.*, p.101
(14)   At this time each Regional Health Authority contained one nursing officer and one public health nursing officer. It should be recognised that while the main body of nursing was controlled by the Ministry of Health, prison nurses and military nurses were outside this control.
(15)   White, *op cit.*, ch.4
(16)   RCNA RCN/T/10. Royal College of Nursing oral transcripts
(17)   *Ibid.*
(18)   RCN/T/10. Royal College of Nursing oral transcripts
(19)   MRC MS/229/CO/4/1/15. COHSE files
(20)   The Royal Medico-Psychological Association handed over the responsibility for the training of psychiatric nurses to the General Nursing Council in 1951, but the GNC's concerns still concentrated on general nurse training.
(21)   The WHO was trying to encourage Britain to place greater emphasis on preventative and community medicine. For a more in-depth study of the WHO nursing policy during this period, see Splane and Splane, *op cit.*
(22)   RCN/T/10. Royal College of Nursing oral transcripts
(23)   Prior to 1948 the Home Office controlled mental health and mental handicap hospitals; a trained nurse was a member of the inspectorate body for these hospitals, but information relating to inspection reports was severely restricted.
(24)   Correspondence between the nursing division of the Ministry of Health and members of the general public reflected the nursing leadership's commitment to mental health. One letter was addressed to the 'Nurse in charge of Britain's sanity'. On her retirement, Dame Elizabeth was asked by the Ministry to work on the Committee of Brookwood Mental Hospital.
(25)   The first outpatient scheme for the mentally ill was initiated by the Cassell Trust with money donated by Sir Felix Cassell. Dame Elizabeth Cockayne served on the Board of Trustees.
(26)   White, *op cit.*

(27)   As CNO, Dame Elizabeth Cockayne experienced considerable difficulties with members of her own profession. It has been assumed that nurses 'entered the NHS like crusaders' (White, *op. cit.*) but this was clearly not the case. Many nurses resented the imposition of the NHS, objected to the end of voluntary hospitals and entered the NHS with trepidation. The Queen's Institute for District Nurses, which was 'a rather superior body' (RCN/T/10, Royal College of Nursing oral transcripts), threatened nurses with dismissal if they worked directly for a local authority not affiliated to the Institute. Furthermore, Institute nurses refused to accept that, as a result of NHS reforms, local authorities controlled district nurse training. Institute objections were only stifled following lengthy negotiations.

(28)   The nursing establishment is represented by the GNC, the RCN and the AHM.

(29)   According to Dame Kathleen, the Salmon enquiry was a direct result of her visit to America, although the moves to initiate the administrative reorganisation of nursing coincided with government concerns over existing administrative inefficiency within the NHS as a whole.

(30)   RCNA K RCN/T/30. Raven, oral history transcript, 1988.

(31)   K. Raven in *International History of Nursing Journal*, 1 no. 2 (1995), p.68

(32)   Clay, *op. cit.*

(33)   The recommendations of the 1972 report into the nursing service, chaired by Professor Asa Briggs, were used as the foundation for the current Project 2000 method of nurse training.

(34)   Raven, *op cit.*

(35)   *COHSE Journal*, March/April 1963: extract from a 1,000-word document in support of a Royal Commission of Enquiry into nursing problems, presented to Congress House on 18th March 1962.

(36)   *COHSE Journal*, January/February 1958, p.17. The Ministry of Health stated that 70% of all student nurses abandoned training within the first year.

(37)   Military service is also underpinned by strong associations with royalty and religion. In fact, most religious services within military realms include the hymn 'Fight the Good Fight' and the official military salute is directed at the Queen's Commission rather than towards an individual officer.

(38)   MRC MSS/229/6/HA/3/1/15. A quote from Will Hayden, Secretary of the National Union of Public Employees, Guildford Hospital Branch.

(39)   This situation represented a break in the chain of command in the military sense and explains to some extent why civilian nurses were struggling for a voice in the NHS while military nurses were involved in medical planning arrangements within NATO. British nursing officers were also the highest ranking female officers in Europe. C. Enloe, *Does Khaki Become You?* (1983), p.102-3

(40)   RCNA RCN/4/39. *Bulletin and Scottish Pictorial*, 1st July 1948

(41)   RAMCR RAMC/1/57/259. Wellcome Institute, London.

(42)   *The Lancet*, 17th November 1951, p.935

(43)   G.E. Godber, *British National Health Service* (1976), p.113. Geographic Health Studies Programme, US Department of Health, Education and Welfare NIH 77.1205. Conversations with Sir George Godber.

(44)   *The Lancet*, 17th November 1951, p.396

(45)   *The Daily Telegraph*, 15th November 1949

(46)   *Liverpool Daily Post*, 15th November 1949

(47)   *British Medical Journal*, 3rd December 1949, p.14

(48)   RCN/4/39

(49)   The medical minutes examined have concentrated on London, Oxford and Bristol hospitals. However, oral history tapes of nursing officers working in Manchester during the 1960s suggest that a similar view was held by doctors in the north of Britain.

(50)   *Journal of British Nursing*, editorial, August 1950, p.1

(51)   RCNA RCN/17/2/2. Letter from Mrs Bennett at the Ministry of Labour to Frances Goodall, Secretary of the Royal College of Nursing.

(52)   *Ibid.*

(53)   *Ibid.*

(54)   In 1947 the GNC received a letter from the Registered Nurses Association in British Columbia cancelling reciprocal arrangements with Britain.

(55)   *Journal of British Nursing*, July 1950. p.87

(56) *News and Times Worcester*, 7th October 1953, and *London Observer*, 9th October 1953 (my emphasis). See also RCN/17/4/39. The original date for launching the educational appeal was 1946 but it was thought that this would detract from the 'British Empire War Memorial Fund'. The educational appeal was therefore postponed until 1950.

(57) Meeting of the *Nursing Times* Advisory Board, July 1960.

(58) *Ibid.*

(59) RCNA RCN/2/2. Report of the RCN Nursing Research Council, January 1960.

(60) Dingwall et.al, p.205-6. Bedford Fenwick had advocated a nursing curriculum organised along medical lines.

(61) RCNA RCN/8/2. N. Mackenzie, extract from a series of lectures given between December 1953 and January 1954.

(62) RCNA RCN/2/2. Report of the RCN Research Council, January 1960.

(63) MRC MSS229/6/C/CO/7/7I. Brook, oral history interview, 27th October 1982.

(64) MRC MSS299/6/C/HA/3/1/1-27. News coverage of Hyde Park demonstration, 16th August 1948.

(65) MRC MSS229/6/C/CO/7/20D. Westmacott, oral history interview, 25th April 1979.

(66) MRC MSS229/CO/4/1/12. Report of 1958 COHSE annual conference.

(67) The RCN became a union in 1977 but was included from 1948 onwards in pay negotiations via Whitley Council machinery.

(68) Pay disputes are examined in more depth in Chapter 7 dealing with political protest.

(69) RCN/7/7/10/2. Letter to the Ministry of Health from the RCN, 7th April 1966.

(70) MRC MSS229/CO/4/1/15. COHSE files

(71) MRC *COHSE Journal*, November/December 1958, p.12

(72) The Horder report is dealt with in Chapter 1

(73) Clay, *op cit.*, p.105

(74) MRC *COHSE Journal*, July/August 1961, p.7

(75) Report of a job analysis in The Nuffield Provincial Hospitals Trust, *The Work of Nurses in Hospital Wards*, (1953), p.129

(76) J. Markham, 'From Service to Civilian Practice', unpublished paper given at the Royal College of Nursing 'Legacy of War' conference, 30th May 1995.

(77) Case assignment patients could number between one and ten depending on the severity of a patient's illness.

(78) Nuffield Provincial Hospitals Trust, *op. cit.*, p.141

(79) *Ibid.*

(80) Maclean, *op cit.*, p.105

(81) Titmuss, *op cit.*, p.202

(82) D. Pyke, 'The Work of Guttman in Relation to Paraplegic Patients', unpublished seminar paper given at the Wellcome Institute, Oxford, 1st March 1996.

(83) *British Nursing Journal*, October 1951, editorial.

(84) RCNA RCN/8/2. N. Mackenzie, 'Needs and Resources in the Nursing Profession' (1954), p.6

(85) RCNA RCN/8/2. N. Mackenzie, 'An End in Itself' (1954), p.10. Teaching these social graces became particularly important as the nursing profession believed that girls were using nursing as a means of 'social advancement and improvement'.

(86) RCNA RCN/8/2. N. Mackenzie, 'The Background' (1954), p.8

(87) Patients were still subjected to saline baths in the 1970s, particularly on gynaecological wards.

(88) Titmuss, *op cit.*, p.200

(89) RCNA RCN/13/ED/1. *The Daily Telegraph*, 5th August 1949. The incident took place in the outpatients department of Miller Hospital, Greenwich; the patient was a 32-year old man who worked as a barge trimmer.

(90) This statement is made in relation to civilian nurses. The nurse as technician developed rapidly within the armed forces as nurses were afforded greater legal protection.

(91) Oral history, interview with Colonel E.E. Gruber von Arni, RRC L/QARANC. Millbank, London, October 1993.

(92) Recruitment figures for the military nursing services remained high until the late 1960s when according to military personnel figures dropped s a result of the media coverage given to the Vietnam War.

(93) White, *op cit.*, p.263

Chapter 7

Uniform Attraction

The rejection of educational reform in the immediate post-war period left nurses with little option other than to align themselves with existing authoritarian professions. Since the profession failed to wake up to this problem, stagnation was inevitable. Professional conservatism, however, was significantly challenged by the influx of men into nursing from 1945 onwards, although this challenge was muted for some time by the reluctance of female nurses to fully include their male colleagues in professional negotiations.

It was certainly not a coincidence that, once men were admitted to the RCN in 1960, the profession shifted more confidently in the direction of education. Men were also responsible for the increased levels of militancy during the pay disputes of this period. The impact of male nurses on both these issues signalled a distinct turning point in nursing history since improvements in education and pay were considered essential in terms of underpinning the professional status of the registered nurse. Conflicting definitions of the term 'professionalism', however, continued to restrict nursing development. For some occupational groups the term merely implied a level of competence in the workplace, whereas for others professionalism encompassed a wide range of ethical and intellectual concerns. The medical and legal profession, for instance, underpinned the acquisition of intellectual knowledge with a rigid code of ethics, a 'moral' dimension that enhanced prestige and inspired public confidence far more effectively than traditional credentialist strategies.

Traditional methods of obtaining professional status had centred on exclusionary recruitment policies and prolonged periods of training, designed to restrict access to the professional group. This process incorporated a series of standardised examinations, and credibility was reinforced by state recognition of professional qualifications. In addition, a wide variety of ceremonial rituals were established to indicate symbolic acceptance to the professional group. Despite this tried and tested formula for achieving professional recognition, however, the boundaries which separated a trade from a profession appeared to be movable and ill-defined. According to the Trades Disputes Act of 1906, a trade included all persons employed in trade and industry, a definition which implied that all persons excluded from trade and industry could be viewed as professional. This situation was further complicated by the fact that some professional groups, such as teachers, formed trade unions while many tradesmen established professional organisations and guilds. From 1960 onwards, even the military became a 'professional' institution, terminology that merely reflected the transition from conscripted to voluntary military service.

Most occupational groups were confused by the term 'professionalism'. Many considered that differences between a profession and a trade centred on whether or not a person sold a product instead of time and knowledge. Others divided occupations along manual and non-manual lines. Ironically, given the lack of progression in nursing practice, the *Journal of British Nursing* claimed that:

> *... the difference between a trade and a profession is essentially that the former is a thing which can be learnt once and for all, to be a professional nurse it is essential to be progressive. To be unprogressive is to reduce our work to the level of an ordinary trade.* [1]

Although the Journal was also quick to point out that most nurses upheld the:

> *... methods in vogue in their training school as those which should be employed in perpetuity and look with suspicion upon any more recently introduced, although these may be the inevitable outcome of fuller knowledge.* [2]

This situation was not surprising. The absence of adequate theoretical education left nurses with little alternative but to cling to nursing methods acquired during training. Thus their professional aspirations were effectively curtailed. As Macdonald has observed in his study of the sociology of professions, 'In addition to the knowledge in practice, there must also be an academic version - the formal abstract knowledge system'. [3]

Within the nursing establishment, professional alignment strategies indicated conflicting attitudes towards professionalism, these in turn reflected the entrenched 'character versus intellect' debate. On the one hand, senior nurses involved in nurse education favoured alignment with the teaching profession, while on the other, those involved in clinical practice compared their position with that of the police and prison service. Nurses were also anxious to maintain existing levels of authority within the healthcare system. The introduction of the NHS had in reality undermined this authority at all levels; nurses had responded by reinforcing authoritarian rules and regulations at every opportunity. The foundations of nurse authority had all but disappeared, but the image of nurse authority had assumed unrealistic proportions. As a result of wartime militarisation, the public image of the nurse had shifted dramatically away from that of the 'handmaiden' towards that of the 'battleaxe'.[4] An Australian film entitled *Handmaidens and Battleaxes*, released in 1987, argued that this changing image was due to the fact that nursing had 'been born in the Church but bred in the Army'.[5] Not surprisingly, the majority of nurses viewed this change of image in a favourable light, primarily because the 'battleaxe' implied that nurses were able to exert authority while the 'handmaiden' had suggested subservience to the medical profession.

Subsequently, by strongly identifying with military style authority, the nursing profession had naturally aligned itself with the police force and the prison service rather than the teaching profession. Their position in society reinforced this alignment. Nurses, in conjunction with the police force and prison service, were required to assist the Home Office and the military regarding issues of civil defence',[6] and until 1948 the Home Office controlled not only the police force and the prison service but also the administration of mental health nursing. The Ministry of Health assumed responsibility for the mentally ill in 1948 but, because of the exclusionary policies pursued by the RCN, a proportion of male nurses working within this field retained their membership of the Prison Officers Union. By the mid 1950s mental health nurses still compared their position in terms of pay and conditions with that of prison officers, while general nurses tended to compare their position with that of police officers.

As uniformed public service personnel, nurses, police and prison officers shared similar work patterns, recruitment problems and military traditions. They adopted and transmitted 'acceptable' values within society and, as such, were responsible for aspects of social control. More importantly, the existence of shared 'acceptable values' provided a structural belief system which fostered professional alignment between these groups.

Evidently, nurses did not make concerted efforts to realign occupational interests. But, although visible realignment did not occur, there appeared to be a general trend towards greater radicalism when dealing with pay disputes. During the 1960s nurses initiated two major confrontations with the Treasury: the first of these occurred in 1962 when nurses opposed the Conservative Government's 'pay pause', and the second in 1969 as nurses challenged the Labour Government's 'prices and incomes' policy. Nevertheless, while the latter dispute was more virulent than the former, this did not indicate a new political cohesion within nursing.

The high profile 'Raise the Roof' campaign, for instance, which began in 1969, was orchestrated by the public relations manager for the RCN, Colonel Douglas de Cent. Campaigners argued that by 'raising the roof' instead of conforming to 'pay ceilings', the salaries of all healthcare workers would be improved. However, it was the absence of adequate pay differentials between registered and ancillary grade nurses that provided the motivating force for radical action. The radicalism displayed by registered nurses, therefore, was not designed to benefit all grades of nursing. Political protest merely provided an opportunity to reassert the status of the registered nurse above 'other ranks'. Although nursing did experience a shift to the left in terms of political affiliations, this move coexisted with attempts to reinforce the boundaries of military style authority. An analysis of pay campaigns is provided in Chapter 8. Firstly, however, in order to understand the professional ambitions associated with these pay campaigns, it is helpful to examine the differences and similarities which existed with the uniformed public services.

Uniformed public services in civil society have traditionally exhibited military influence. Police, nurses, prison officers and firemen all incorporated military values and organisational structures. Members of these services were recruited primarily from the middle classes in order to maintain an affinity between service values and the values of the ruling classes. These links between military and civil society were further strengthened by the fact that ex-military personnel were frequently drawn to civilian public service, as highlighted by the following statements obtained from police recruits:

> *I have a lot to offer the service and the community. I have ten years' experience in the Army to draw upon and I am used to the discipline and wearing of uniform.*

> *At present I am serving in the Royal Navy as a Leading Regulator. I want to carry on in uniformed service. The police is an ideal second career for me.*

> *I was a supervisor in the military police but the people I went for a drink with, that I talked to and related to, were civil police officers, mainly CID.*

> *I see myself helping the community by leadership, gaining the respect of children by setting a good example so that they can base their lives on this example.* [7]

Military and civilian links were made explicit with regard to police discipline and uniform, but recruits also considered value systems to be important. Gaining community respect and status by transmitting certain values and providing exemplary leadership were recurrent themes in all uniformed public service recruits. There was also a notion that recruits needed to possess a sense of vocation and duty, although this same 'vocational spirit' argument continually worked against recruits since it was often used to negate pay claims. Senior members of the nursing profession, for instance, maintained that high salaries would attract the 'wrong' kind of girl into the profession. This view was echoed by a Home Office report into the recruitment of people with higher educational qualifications into the police service. The 1967 report proclaimed that:

> *Anyone contemplating a career in the police service must be predisposed towards public service and no public service can seriously compete with private industry to attract the man whose principal concern is to make as much money as he can. Nor is such a person likely to make an ideal recruit to the police.* [8]

Similarly, the police service suffered from the character versus intellect debate in much the same way as the nursing services. The public impression of the police was that of a 'service which had little interest in attracting brains'.[9]

Along with members of the ambulance service, police officers and nurses were held in high esteem within individual communities. The general public appeared to recognise the vocational content of these employment fields and placed its members on a pedestal in relation to other occupations. This level of prestige provided an incentive to recruitment, despite the fact that members of the uniformed public services were always in danger of falling off their pedestal, particularly when pay disputes were in the offing. Due to a combination of government wage restraints and the need to provide a twenty-four hour nursing service, most nurses were expected to work long hours for little reward. When nurses pressed for improved working conditions, however, they frequently met with public disapproval. The desire to retain public trust acted as a barrier to radical action and vocational arguments were continually used to undermine pay demands. Eventually, the recruitment incentive of being afforded a high status within society was far outweighed by the recruitment deterrent of having to endure poor working conditions. In this context the essential question is not why these services experienced recruitment problems, but why anyone would want to be employed in uniformed public service in the first instance.

Many recruits were attracted by the benefits associated with uniformed service. For example, employees enjoyed subsidised accommodation and food, free laundry facilities and room cleaning. These net advantages mirrored the institutional lifestyle of the armed forces, and ex-military staff experienced these professions as a 'home from home'. The existence of military-style uniforms reinforced this position. Similarly, a sense of group loyalty and cohesion was fostered within the police, prison and nursing services in much the same manner as in military regiments.[10] A process of formal occupational socialisation encouraged *'esprit de corps'* and informal cultural experiences ensured vertical integration within the individual organisations. Training was primarily geared towards reducing diversity and producing collective thinking. Emphasis was also placed on personal character building and orientation to rule-based regimes. With regard to social values, existing attitudes of recruits were systematically moulded in order to endorse the class bias of the state - a process which did not normally present a problem since recruits were mainly drawn from middle-class backgrounds.

Although new recruits were attracted by support networks and a sense of camaraderie, undoubtedly the biggest attraction for some lay with the uniform itself. Most described their uniform as a symbol of legitimate authority, commanding automatic respect from members of the general public. Promotions were marked by changes in uniform and status conveyed through symbolic deference to the levels of hierarchy. Nevertheless, while the public recognised the authority associated with individual uniforms, outward signs of status were aimed primarily at reinforcing institutional security and group identity. As Salvage has pointed out, nursing was 'notoriously status-conscious' and loved the trappings of uniform.[11] Ranks were denoted by stripes on hats and sleeves, the wearing of badges, different coloured dresses and belts and varying styles of caps, aprons and starched cuffs. Much of this symbolism was wasted on patients, to whom nurses were all those dressed in a white cap and apron. Public reactions to the police were similar; while people recognised the overall uniform, they did not necessarily appreciate the distinctions between hierarchical levels. The symbolic trappings of authority may have given satisfaction to those wearing the uniforms, but they were not required for public recognition.

In reality, the preoccupation with rank was largely indicative of professional insecurity which, in turn, fostered a desire to establish hierarchies within the profession. This lack of professional confidence was directly related to the lack of adequate academic knowledge since 'on the job' training methods were favoured above formal teaching techniques. Whereas it can be argued that these methods were still appropriate for the fire and ambulance services, they were less so for the police, nursing and prison services. This was partly due to their differing roles. Fire and ambulance services were primarily concerned with immediacy of action for a limited time period, whereas nurses, police and prison officers were involved in community action on a long-term basis - they were concerned with the ongoing wellbeing of patients and prisoners. Police and nurses in particular maintained a high profile within society and came into contact with the general public far more than any other occupational group. Nevertheless, all three services were handicapped by the limitations of their training. The uniform often added an extra burden since people tended to become more mechanised and less human when wearing a uniform denoting authority. As Howard observed with regard to the prison service, 'for people whose work in the future must be primarily devoted to bridging a gap between themselves and men of particularly unstable social behaviour, a uniform is a distinct handicap'.[12] A similar position arose in the hospital setting whereby some patients were intimidated by the air of brisk efficiency associated with a nurse's uniform.

However, although issues of status dominated the concerns of nurses, prison officers and police, only the latter group confronted professional insecurity with positive action. Experimental measures were first introduced in 1934 when Lord Trenchard as Police Commissioner (formerly of the RAF) decided that the force lacked effective leadership. In an attempt to create military-style officer material, Trenchard established a Metropolitan Police College at Hendon which was later disbanded with the outbreak of war in 1939. In stark contrast to the nursing profession, the Hendon scheme had met with considerable opposition from within the force because of its elitism:

It was regarded as a deliberate attempt to create an officer class structure in the police service with higher posts reserved for a privileged elite. [13]

Despite its elitism, the Hendon experiment was considered a success in terms of providing leadership, and once the war was over a National Police College was established at Bramshill. Whereas the Hendon scheme had concentrated on man management, Bramshill incorporated a broader knowledge base in subjects such as forensic science.

More importantly, Bramshill managed to gain the approval of the Police Federation. While nurses were busy constructing a class-based elite, the police were making moves towards a system of promotion by means of meritocracy. A more egalitarian attitude could also be detected in the treatment of constables.

During the 1930s a special class of constable was introduced into the force, recruited on a short-term basis with no promotional opportunities whatsoever. The Police Federation argued that this policy was discriminatory and senior positions should not be reserved for certain classes of entrants. The position of special class constable, therefore, was duly abandoned. This situation had direct parallels with the position of the State Enrolled Assistant Nurse within the nursing hierarchy, who was also unable to obtain promotion, unlike the special class constable. However, the SEAN continued to suffer discrimination.

The Police Federation had confronted class elitism and an anti-intellectual bias to some extent, but these problems were not totally eradicated. Recruits remained overwhelmingly middle-class and, despite the growing population of blacks and Asians, these groups were rarely incorporated into the force. With regard to intellectualism, Bramshill had provided university scholarships for outstanding recruits and in 1967 twenty-one such scholarships were awarded. In addition, many forces made arrangements to send senior officers on university courses. In terms of graduate intake, however, recruitment was not particularly impressive. Between 1945 and 1965, only twenty-five out of a possible half a million graduates entered the force[14] and the majority of police recruits were accepted without any qualifications. This picture resembled the recruitment patterns of the prison and nursing services.

By 1960 it was evident that all three services were failing to attract recruits of high intellectual ability. The police fared better than nurses and prison officers because they had managed to retain control of their professional interests. The intellectually demanding aspects of the prison service, such as welfare, rehabilitation, education and probation work, were eventually established as separate professions. Nurses experienced a similar decline, losing control of radiography, physiotherapy and occupational therapy. In contrast, the police retained control of a myriad of employment sections that were usually linked to district centres. This process was assisted by the division of the police force into uniformed and non-uniformed branches.

Since nurses and prison officers had failed to extend their fields of influence, they were left with the most mundane of jobs. This trend could not be reversed without new attitudes to professional development. As the Confederation of Health Service Employees pointed out:

> *Matrons need new thinking and a change in leadership if they are to continue, for as sure as day follows night the matrons will soon find others prepared to carry out administrative functions.* [15]

But as part of the military legacy matrons had been intent on maintaining fruitless, time-consuming ward inspections and had steadfastly refused to assume new responsibilities. A similar military legacy was active within the prison service where, in addition to conforming to rigid rules, junior members were required to salute senior staff.[16] These practices became increasingly open to criticism. As Howard noted in 1960:

> *It should be as ludicrous for a prison officer to salute his governor in the institutions of the future as it would be now for a psychiatric social worker to salute her psychiatrist before getting down to discussion of case histories with him.* [17]

Undoubtedly, the prison service was excessively militarised. Prison Commissioners resembled military commanders who were remote from the ordinary workforce and operated in much the same way as a military headquarters.

The effects of militarisation were explicit within all uniformed public service, and it is difficult to assess how these services would have developed in the absence of military influence. Howard has argued that the work of Prison Commissioners needed to resemble that of the Inspectorate of Education since, in the field of education, inspectors were not distanced from the main workforce and there was less pomp and ceremony attached to official visits, whereas, with regard to the police service, Brogden has claimed that problems originated with a lack of government control as official investigations into police organisation reinforced the authority of police chiefs rather than that of the Home Office.[18] By comparison, nurses had very little authority, even though they managed to present an image of being in control at all times. Without military influence, prison officers and nurses may have recognised the need for intellectual knowledge at an earlier stage. Given this recognition, professions such as occupational therapy may have developed as branches of nursing. However, it was not merely the anti-educational bias which provided an obstacle to change. The process of moulding the attitudes of new recruits prevented wide-scale experimentation. While other professions incorporated liberal thinkers, police, nurses and prison officers were indoctrinated into military value systems which increasingly bore little relation to a rapidly changing civilian society.

This indoctrination process supported the idea of British supremacy over other nationalities and stressed the importance of historical traditions. In addition, recruits were encouraged to adopt a sense of duty and the moral high ground in their dealings with the public. Within nursing spheres these values were conveyed more by continuous suggestion at ward level than by direct tuition in the classroom. The justification for such indoctrination varied between the services. Nora Mackenzie, a nurse educationalist, explained that since many new recruits were idealistic in nature they needed to be protected from disillusionment: 'We have a responsibility to see that the ideals and sense of values with which they arrive are not lost by their new contacts'.[19] There was also the notion that nurses were required to accept existing working conditions along with existing values. As Mackenzie further stated, 'we know that more ought to be done but we must accept with a quiet spirit what can be done'.[20] Within the police, value systems were essential for maintaining an occupational framework by which to judge individual criminal actions. There was also the desire to protect police work from public criticism. Reuss-Ianni's analysis of street and management policing methods revealed that 'everyone in the department was socialised to this ethos, the values of loyalty and privilege and the importance of keeping department business inside the department'.[21] The situation differed yet again within the prison service. Here, values were transmitted in a more overtly military style and were considered vital for ensuring control of prisoner activities. As Howard observed:

The best of the older prison officers adopt towards the young assistant governor an attitude rather like that of a good sergeant major in the army towards a newly commissioned subaltern. [22]

The key reasons for the indoctrination process, however, centred on the need to maintain control not only over the general public but also over members of staff. This fundamental process ensured that uniformed public service could never be equated with more liberal based professions.

The Paradox of Control

Throughout the 1950s, at least the uniformed services appeared to provide a bastion of social control, defending the values which were assumed to have played an important role in establishing the British Empire. This was a period characterised by an increasing concern for civil defence in the climate of cold war politics when many ordinary civilians volunteered to join civil defence forces, although more volunteers were motivated by the privileged car parking facilities afforded to civil defence force members than by a genuine fear of foreign aggression. However, military personnel, nurses, prison officers and the police viewed the issue of civil defence in a more sombre light. Systematic lectures were given on how to care for casualties in the event of nuclear war and the co-ordination of civil military medical planning. Subsequently, the civilian services adopted a military style language. Nurses and police were taught at all times to convey complete reassurance to the general public and to remain calm in all situations. For example, in the treatment of psychiatric casualties of nuclear war, medical personnel were advised to be extremely careful in using terminology:

> *Terms such as neurosis, neurasthenia, nervous breakdown, mental shock should be avoided and replaced by expressions like fatigue or exhaustion, conveying the impression of a condition which a good night's sleep will soon put right.* [23]

Despite the fact that both military and civilian personnel knew very little about the effects of nuclear war, this fact was not widely appreciated by members of the public. The uniformed services occupied a position of trust within society, and in order to retain this trust the military relied on secrecy of action. Military personnel assumed an air of authority in all situations and mistakes in military strategy were concealed whenever possible. This process served to reinforce the illusion of military efficiency which subsequently influenced civilian industry and public service alike. Intense militarisation of civilian nursing in the 1950s ran parallel to the militarisation of the police force. Both professions adopted a similar military stance in their dealings with the general public, and the social control of the civilian population was achieved largely by a process of bluff. Though the social controls which were exerted on the private lives of members of uniformed public services far outweighed the strictures of normal civilian employment fields. In practice civilian nurses were expected to adhere to stricter disciplinary codes than those imposed on their military colleagues. The police force suffered from a similar experience, although there was considerable public resistance to the 'restoration of a Blimpish controlled, military ranked force which contrasted unfavourably with the work of auxiliaries during the war'.[24]

Despite the fact that nurses and police exerted social control along military lines, they were paradoxically subjected to greater controls than the remainder of the population. By endorsing military style organisation, both professions appeared to automatically adopt some of the social aspects of military life. For instance, it was common practice within military circles to exercise control over the off-duty time of personnel. This practice was duly incorporated into the civilian police, prison and nursing services. The rules and regulations that extended into the private lives of police and nurses in particular were extraordinarily petty. A policeman's wife, for example, was not allowed to open a shop or business near her husband's place of work, while a registered nurse was not allowed to fraternise with junior members of staff. Therefore, although nurses and police officers were able to exert more authority than those employed in other occupational fields, this ability resulted in a corresponding loss of personal liberty.

It was precisely this paradox of control that created tension within the nursing service and the police force. Difficulties associated with recruitment and high wastage rates within these occupations indicated that members resented the petty restrictions which governed their private lives. More liberal attitudes within civilian society had also undermined the process of moulding recruits. By 1960, the military model of nursing organisation was becoming increasingly anachronistic and existing training methods were not achieving the cohesive compliant workforce of previous years.

The shift towards more liberal societal attitudes was not dramatic however. Capital punishment was still in force until 1965 and the Equal Pay Act was not introduced until 1970. Despite the fact that racial discrimination had emerged as an important political issue, the 1968 Commonwealth Immigration Act was still overtly racist in nature. Nevertheless, there was a growing recognition by some members of society that traditional values needed to be questioned. The wellspring of liberal attitudes originated with members of the intelligentsia and some sections of middle-class Britain, but they were not always helpful in producing change. As Tony Benn recalled, responses to papers discussing the problems of race relations did not usually provoke radical action. 'Reaction was rather typically liberal middle-class, feeling that to stress race as an issue was to accentuate differences which morally ought not to exist'.[25]

However, if middle-class liberalism was not entirely helpful in resolving racial problems, there was at least a recognition that racism was inextricably linked to the class system. If British society intended to maintain a racial hierarchy then immigrants needed to be confined to the lower sections of the social hierarchy. Racial conflict was also more prevalent in areas where this hierarchy was not well defined. In many respects this was not surprising; the notion of British racial superiority was a legacy of the Empire and ingrained within the fabric of both military and civilian society. Certainly, many immigrants were unskilled workers, but there were others who were highly skilled professionals. Subsequently, within the field of healthcare delivery, notions of racial superiority conflicted with the need to rely on immigrant doctors to staff the NHS. Nurses who attempted to maintain the idea of racial superiority by restricting registration courses to white middle-class girls were simultaneously subordinated to orders issued by immigrant doctors. Between 1950 and 1960 there was an increase of 4,000 doctors employed in the health service, and 3,000 of this total were from overseas.[26] Clearly, the NHS depended on the services of immigrant doctors, dentists and other professionals who were not content to be relegated to the lower realms of social hierarchy.

The process of rethinking racial attitudes ran parallel to changing attitudes regarding education. The 1960s were characterised by a move towards meritocracy, motivated by notions of egalitarianism within government administration and by technological changes in industry and commerce. Traditional promotion strategies had relied on the military style time promotion theory,[27] based on an assumption that over a certain period of time a person should have accumulated enough experience to move upwards onto the next rung of the career ladder. This process did not always involve the acquisition of new knowledge. Changes in technology and a corresponding demand for greater intellectual knowledge resulted in more specialist courses in all fields of employment. Moreover, while this process was partly due to the growth of new professions such as public relations, it nevertheless reflected a shift away from practical training techniques; thus experience and social character no longer claimed total precedence over intellectual knowledge. Albeit a gradual transition, civilian society was gravitating towards liberalism and rejecting long-standing military values.

Responses to this transition varied within professional circles. Some professionals agitated for progress and reform while others resisted change at all costs. Teachers, for instance, had stressed the need for changes in the vocational guidance given to young girls, since the International Labour Conference of 1949 had declared that, although guidance should be geared towards making individuals aware of their special aptitudes, it should also steer girls in the direction of careers in the home. In response, The *Woman Teacher* journal pointed out that 'it was dangerous and wrong that a specific occupation should be singled out in this way as one which girls should be made aware'.[28] The *Woman Teacher* also drew attention to the fact that the *British Medical Journal* refused to accept advertisements for medical officers if salaries offered varied depending on whether applicants were male or female. This policy, they argued, should be adopted by the teaching profession as part of the wider campaign for equal pay. However, the Campaign for Equal Pay, which had achieved considerable support during the war, was somewhat delayed in the post-war years by the amalgamation of women's unions with men's. As Walby has demonstrated, this process led to a 'serious decline in the representation of the interests of women workers'.[29] Nevertheless, women teachers were in the forefront of the battle for equal pay, along with local government officers and civil servants.

Female nurses found themselves in an untenable position with regard to sexual discrimination. The RCN offered token support to the equal pay campaign while simultaneously preventing men from joining the College. As demonstrated in Chapter 3, various methods were deployed to block male entry into the field of general nursing and, once equal pay for nurses was agreed in 1955, nursing support for the broad equal pay movement dwindled. Within the police force, sex differentiation in terms of salaries was reflected by a 9:10 ratio throughout the service and female police officers did not appear to push for equal pay. A Royal Commission in 1960 had received no complaints regarding the issue and therefore continued the 9:10 ratio. Female prison officers, however, fared better than their colleagues in the police; differentials in pay between men and women in the prison service were gradually eliminated from 1955 onwards as a result of an equal pay agreement negotiated by civil service unions. This agreement was phased in over a period of seven years and afforded equal pay to non-industrial civil servants. The negotiating machinery of the civil service did not, however, extend to female police officers.

The civil service frequently set the pace for overall pay demands in other employment areas.[30] Despite the campaign for equal pay, however, women were usually relegated to lower-paid jobs and, in manufacturing industry, women's wages as a proportion of male earnings had not changed significantly from the inter-war period until 1970, although there were some changes in the relationship between skilled and unskilled workers in that the gap between earnings in these groups had widened. The salaries of some professional groups such as lawyers and managerial staff fell in relation to the wages earned by some skilled workers, and this levelling of incomes had narrowed the gap between middle- and working-class lifestyles. These changes were also accompanied by a decline in industrial profit that was attributed to the growing competition from overseas, the militancy of trade unions and the Labour Government's withdrawal of investment incentive schemes.[31]

Not surprisingly, economic changes had prompted a wave of social change. There was a general rise in the standard of living and a rise in consumerism. Members of all social classes were able to afford expensive items such as cars, and the changing patterns of lifestyle were reflected in patterns of ill health. Diseases associated with poverty, such as tuberculosis, were virtually eradicated, while those associated with affluence, such as heart disease, were on the increase. Expanding networks of welfare provision had reduced poverty levels, while universal secondary school education offered a chance for all children to develop intellectual skills. In addition, the creation of extra universities and technical colleges provided new opportunities for career development and research. Despite these considerable changes, however, the public school system remained intact. As Tony Benn recalled of a school in Abingdon:

> *The headmaster was a retired Lieutenant Colonel and discipline was rigid to a degree. I got the feeling of a completely repressed school in which all the natural irreverence and genius of the children had been stamped out.* [32]

The headmaster was also a firm believer in the need for an elite, and highly suspicious of the Robbins Report which advocated the expansion of education. This stance was typical of a public school ethos which continued to provide cadet training schemes in preparation for the military officer corps.

By 1970, however, the public school sector, along with the uniformed public service, represented the only civilian institutions to endorse militarism, where ceremonial presentations of hospital badges for nurses and good conduct medals for the police continued to reinforce the hierarchy and outdated attitudes towards class and race. Within the remaining sections of British society, military influence had diminished. In the 1950s, with the exception of movements such as the Campaign for Nuclear Disarmament (CND), military methods and organisations were regarded as an efficient model for civilian society. By the mid 1960s there was a considerable backlash against military ideology and new concepts of managerial practice were competing with the traditional military model. In addition, the legitimacy of military and civilian authority within society was called into question by a younger generation.

This shift away from authoritarianism was detected within government circles by 1960. With regard to the police service, conflict arose between MPs who advocated local control and those who supported a move towards central control. Prompted by a need to establish the boundaries of control exerted by Chief Constables, the Royal Commission into the police services in 1962 recommended new rules of accountability. These recommendations were duly incorporated into the Police Bill of 1963 and subsequently the Police Act of 1965. The Home Secretary was given more power over Chief Constables and the ability to initiate local enquiries when necessary. The area of jurisdiction for individual constables was extended from local areas to include all of England and Wales. In addition, the Home Secretary had the responsibility of ensuring police efficiency at all levels.

The societal shift away from authoritarianism was therefore accompanied by an increase in central government control, and the police became more overtly militarised. British civilian police had been used to reinforce the military in Cyprus as early as 1958; however the increasing militarisation of mainland police began in 1966 when individual forces started to purchase surplus army rifles. Growing domestic protest against the existence of American air bases in Britain, problems in Northern Ireland, and the increasing threat of mainland terrorism, culminated in greater co-operation between the armed forces and civilian police. The concept of armed police had become an accepted reality of British policing. As Manwaring-White has noted:

Aggressive policing was replacing the benign image of the old-style policeman and shoot to kill had finally replaced the old idea of a defensive weapon in the hands of the British police. [33]

Clearly, therefore, while the police had confronted the militaristic 'character versus intellect' debate at a relatively early stage, in terms of organisation and aggression the police were more rather than less militarised by 1970.

Nurses, meanwhile, had not yet confronted the 'character versus intellect' debate. Some members of the RCN were pushing for educational reform, which eventually culminated in a government enquiry into the nursing services, chaired by Professor Asa Briggs. The Briggs Report, however, was not published until 1972 and educational reform was not implemented until a much later stage. The Salmon administrative reforms had attempted to introduce managerial concepts into nursing organisation but, as demonstrated in Chapter 3, the implementation of these reforms had reinforced the military style hierarchy. The nursing profession did not endorse the shift towards a more liberal society and, therefore, concerns regarding the moral wellbeing of student nurses resulted in tighter controls in nursing homes. Nursing was, however, in the process of being swamped by other healthcare professions and, since restrictions imposed on radiographers were not as rigid as those imposed on nurses, the latter began to resist excessive discipline. Nevertheless, most nurses still believed in the power and status of the uniform. In order to attract more recruits and to highlight the prestige of individual training schools, many hospitals redesigned existing uniforms - the more elaborate the uniform the higher the status. Some nurses in London teaching hospitals took nearly three quarters of an hour to get dressed, simply because of the amount of detachable buttons, cuffs, frills and complicated hats which were incorporated into the nursing uniform. As an exasperated Sir Godber, Chief Medical Officer, announced to an American audience, 'In Britain we have been 25 years in trying to introduce a standard nurse's uniform. Do you think that is possible? You try'.[34]

Conclusion

The attraction of an elaborate uniform had waned considerably by the late 1960s and the emoluments that had served to encourage recruitment had been discarded. Economic constraints had also reduced the support networks available to nurses. In this respect, the nursing services were demilitarised. However, in terms of racist recruitment policies, anti-intellectualism and regimentation, nurses remained intensely militarised, although both the police and nursing services had gradually abandoned the military concept of time promotion. The Salmon administrative reforms, which were implemented from 1969 onwards, allowed for quicker promotion within the nursing service, and a similar policy was adopted within the police force. As a result of the 1967 government enquiry into the recruitment of people with higher educational qualifications into the police service, time promotion was reduced and, in some cases, abolished. For instance, the period which a constable was required to serve before sitting examinations for promotion was reduced from three years to two, while the more general requirement of serving four years before being eligible for promotion was abolished. The police and nursing services differed, however, in that from 1960 onwards nurses adopted a more radical approach when confronting pay disputes. This move towards radicalism finally broke the traditional nursing mould since, by endorsing radicalism, nurses were forced to abandon their 'pedestal' position within society and, subsequently, the paradox of control.

Endnotes

(1)   *Journal of British Nursing* editorial: 'The Professional Mind', August 1955
(2)   *Ibid.*
(3)   D. Macdonald, *The Sociology of the Professions* (1995), p.164
(4)   M. Baly, 'A history of the Royal College of Nursing History Society'. *International History of Nursing Journal*, 1, no.3, (1996) p.62
(5)   RCN Film Collection, Cavendish Square, London, Australian Broadcasting Company, *Handmaidens and Battleaxes* (1987).
(6)   Nurses became involved in civil defence issues from 1950 onwards.
(7)   N.G. Fielding, *Joining Forces* (1988), p.19, 20, 29, 21
(8)   *Recruitment of People with Higher Educational Qualifications into the Police Service*,. HMSO, (1967). para. 38
(9)   *Ibid.*, para 25
(10)   This situation applied less to ambulance and fire services.
(11)   J. Salvage, *The Politics of Nursing* (1985) p.30
(12)   D.L. Howard, *The English Prisons.* (1960)
(13)   *Recruitment of People with Higher Educational Qualifications into the Police Service*, HMSO, (1967) para. 15
(14)   T.A. Critchley, *A History of the Police in England and Wales* (1967) p.304
(15)   MRC MS229/CO/4/1/15. *COHSE Journal*, November/December 1963
(16)   The police were also required to salute senior officers, whereas nurses demonstrated deference in other ways, which are highlighted in Chapter 9.
(17)   Howard, *op cit.*, p.157
(18)   M. Brogden, *The Police Autonomy and Consent* (1982) p.104
(19)   Mackenzie (1954), *op cit.*
(20)   RCNA, RCN/8/2. N. Mackenzie, *Imperatives of Prudence and Management'.* (1953)
(21)   E Reuss-Ianni, *Two Cultures of Policing.* London, 1983
(22)   Howard, *op cit.*
(23)   Wellcome Institute Library, London, RAMC/176/10, p.31
(24)   Brogden, *op cit.*, p.103
(25)   T. Benn, *Out of the Wilderness: diaries 1963-1967* (1987) p.64
(26)   *Parliamentary Debates* (House of Commons) 5th ser.,1962, col.1093
(27)   Except for the most senior of positions, time promotion is still operational within the military.
(28)   *The Woman Teacher*, 30th September 1949, p.234
(29)   S. Walby, *Patriarchy at Work* (University of Minnesota Press, 1986) p.214
(30)   Universities introduced equal pay scales before the Treasury took a lead in this area.
(31)   A. Glyn and B. Sutcliffe, 'The collapse of UK profits' *New Left Review*, (March/April 1971), Investment incentives were withdrawn in the late 1960s.
(32)   Benn, *op cit.*, p.93
(33)   S. Manwaring-White, *The Policing Revolution*, (1983) p.119
(34)   G. Godber, *The British National Health Service: conversations with Sir George Godber* (Washington, 1976) p.88

Chapter 8

Breaking the Mould

Nurses were not traditionally renowned for adopting a militant approach towards salary negotiations. Yet nursing policy regarding pay disputes changed markedly over a relatively short period of time. Major nursing confrontations with Treasury policy occurred in 1962 and 1969. In 1962 nurses retained their 'angel of mercy' image and relied heavily on public sympathy plus support from individual Members of Parliament. But in 1969 nurses were prepared to relinquish their 'angel' image and alienate the public in the process. During both these pay campaigns the aims were identical: firstly, to achieve a reasonable salary in comparison to other professions; and secondly, to reassert the status of the registered nurse above other nursing ranks. While nurses undoubtedly compared their pay scales with those of the police, prison service and the teaching profession, the motivating force for action always stemmed from a lack of adequate pay differentials between trained and untrained nursing staff.

The major nursing disputes were initiated against a backdrop of economic instability. Successive British governments had pursued a 'stop-go' economic policy and, as Table 8.1 demonstrates, this policy did not always have the co-operation of trade unions. Both the pay pause (introduced by the Conservative Government in 1961) and the restraint exercised by the National Prices and Incomes Board (a Labour Government initiative following their election in 1964) signalled 'stop' periods, yet these were the periods when nurses agitated for salary increases. Both pay campaigns were also designed to attract public sympathy, although the Secretary of State for Scotland remarked of the 1962 pay campaign that 'it would be folly to yield to one's emotions and so stimulate another inflationary spiral in which the very people whose case was being pleaded would suffer the most'.[1]

Traditionally, nurses had always appealed for public support when making salary claims and continued to do so irrespective of changes in the negotiating framework. National pay scales, along with Whitley Council negotiating machinery to determine nurse salary increases, emerged with the NHS based on a similar system of Councils already in operation within the civil service. The Nurses and Midwives Whitley Council, like others, was divided into staff and management sides. The staff side comprised of professional and union representatives while the management side comprised of members drawn from

Table 8.1 Summary of wage controls, 1945-79

Period of policy	Name of policy	Govern-ment[a]	Type of policy[b]	TUC cooperation[c]	Enforcing agency	Norm for wage increases (£ per week or annual % change)	Annual percentage change in weekly wage rates:			Associated conditions/concessions
							preceding 6 months	during policy	succeeding 6 months	
07/45-02/48	Postwar restraint	Lab	VC	Yes	TUC	None	..	4.6	3.9	Some market flexibility
02/48-10/50	Cripps-TUC	Lab	VC	Yes	None	None	5.9	2.5	13	Controlled goods' prices frozen; FBI voluntary price/profits restraint
1956	Pay/price plateau	Cons	VC	No	None	None	13.2	1.4	9.7	Productivity deals
07/61-03/62	Selwyn Lloyd's pay pause	Cons	VC	No	None	Zero	1.6	3.6	4.1	None
04/62-10/64	Guiding light	Cons	VC	No	National Incomes Commission	2-2.5% (later 3.5%)	4.8	3.9	4.3	Part of indicative planning exercise
12/64-07/66	Statement of intent	Lab	VC	Yes	National Board for Prices and Incomes	3-3.5%	2.9	5	1.4	Part of indicative planning exercise
07/66-12/66	Freeze	Lab	SC	A	National Board for Prices and Incomes	Zero	4.3	0.2	3.9	
01/67-06/67	Severe restraint	Lab	SC	A	National Board for Prices and Incomes	Zero norm	1.4	3.1	7.9	
06/67-04/68	Relaxation	Lab	SC	A	National Board for Prices and Incomes	3.5	3.9	8.3	3.1	
04/68-06/70	Jenkins: renewed restraint	Lab	SC	HC	None	4.5	7.4	7	16	Abandonment of 'In place of strife'
11/72-03/73	Stage I freeze	Cons	SC	HC	Pay Board Price Commission	Zero	21.4	3.7	19.5	Effective implementation of Industrial Relations Act, 1971
04/73-11/73	Stage II	Cons	SC	HC	Pay Board Price Commission	5.5	8.6	13.5	16.7	Subsidies to state industries
11/73-02/74	Stage III	Cons	SC	HC	Pay Board Price Commission	7% plus partial indexation Indexed to RPI	13.9	12.1	35.6	
03/74-07/74	Social contract I	Lab	VC	Yes	None		10.8	35.2	30.5	Social contract
08/75-07/76	Social contract II	Lab	CC	Yes	None	£6.00 flat rate	31	19.6	4.4	Renewed social contract
08/76-07/77	Social contract III	Lab	CC	Yes	None	£2.50-£4.00	12.3	5.2	7.4	Tax reductions
08/77-07/78	Social contract IV	Lab	CC	Yes	None	10	4.8	17.2	9.4	
08/78-05/79	Social contract V	Lab	CC	No	Clegg commission	5	25.2	12.7	18.1	

Notes:

[a] Lab=Labour; Cons=Conservative. b CC = Compulsory controls; VC = Voluntary controls; SC=Compulsory controls. c A=Acquiescence; HC=Hostile compliance.

Source: Middleton, op. cit., table 12.2.

Regional Health Boards, Hospital Management Committees and five government representatives. Yet the negotiating techniques exhibited by nurses and representatives of the staff side contained strong emotional overtones. During one of the first meetings of the Whitley Council, a report was presented regarding the nursing of the chronic sick. The report, written by Professor Thomson, was circulated at the request of the National Union of Public Employees (NUPE) and made an emotional appeal for better conditions and salaries for nurses working in these areas. Highlighting the appalling working conditions, Professor Thomson stated that:

> *In their quiet endurance and their efficiency, as in their triumph over discouraging circumstances and lack of proper equipment, the nurses recalled the virtues of their fathers in the rank and file of the county regiments who held the trenches in Flanders in the campaign of 1914-18 and saved Europe.* [2]

Rhetoric of this kind enabled nurses to maintain a dignified stance when discussing pay issues. However, negotiations which centred on a sense of nurse martyrdom ultimately undermined the validity of nurse pay claims. Nurses were adopted the role of victim, encouraging public sympathy by adhering to the 'angel' image but failing to stress their right to fair remuneration simply on the basis of being a professional body. As one member of the opposition stated in the House of Commons in 1962, 'I think the memory of Florence Nightingale has done more to damage the living standards of staff in the National Health Service than anything else'.[3] The sense of nurse martyrdom continued, however, albeit somewhat subdued by the 1960s. In a letter to *The Times* in 1962, Catherine Hall, the General Secretary of the RCN, appealed to the public to support nurse pay claims. The letter, published a week before a marathon parliamentary debate on the issue, stated that:

> *The professional ethics of nurses and midwives preclude action detrimental to the service they give to the community; but it would be contrary to the British sense of justice to allow further exploitation of this spirit of service.* [4]

These public appeals, coupled with the lobbying of MPs, did achieve a certain degree of success. While the House of Commons debated the issue of nurse pay claims on 27th March 1962, the length of the discussion clearly indicated substantial support for nurses. The debate continued throughout the night for a period of nearly thirteen hours and was described by one MP as an emotional attack on the government. The debate also reflected wider dissatisfaction with

Conservative economic policy. In accordance with the government's 'pay pause', all healthcare professionals were offered a blanket 2.5% pay rise. These included almoners, physiotherapists, psychiatric social workers and nurses. Even biochemists and physicians were offered the same amount, despite the fact that they had requested similar rates to their counterparts in the government scientific service.

Professional salaries generally had lagged behind the increases awarded to wage earners, but nursing salaries had suffered the most. A police constable, for instance, received a starting pay of £12 per week plus 42s rent allowance. Radiographers were able to earn £11 a week within the NHS or £17 in the private sector. Even a typist was able to earn £15 per week and a secretary £16 per week. In comparison, a male nurse received a weekly salary of £8.13s.4d. The differentials between civilian and military nursing had also widened considerably. In 1947 military nurses had a £46 per year lead over civilian nurses; by 1962 this lead had escalated to the sum of £239. Not surprisingly, many nurses were flocking to join the armed forces or leaving Britain to nurse in the USA and Canada. Registered nurses in Canada were able to earn £1,213 per annum, rising to £1,376 with three years' service, compared to £525 per annum rising to £656 after six years' service in Britain. However, the real indignation for registered nurses centred on the fact that, with overtime rates, ward orderlies were earning far more than qualified staff. There were also pay anomalies across nursing fields. Nurses in the mental field were paid overtime, but nurses in the general field were not, thus a registered nurse with twenty-five years' service could earn £11.13s.3d a week while a ward orderly with less than six weeks' experience could earn £13 a week.

Nevertheless, as ministers debated the issue of nurse pay it was clear that many still believed in the vocational spirit of nursing. If pay increases were substantial, they argued, the 'wrong' type of girl would enter the profession and, as Enoch Powell, Minister of Health, argued, it was not as though the government expected nurses to comply with rules which did not apply to the rest of the nation. Everyone in industry and public service was required to adhere to the 'pay pause'. Members of the opposition pointed out, however, there were considerable grounds for making nurses a special case; they further argued that the vocational argument no longer applied since many nurses were now 'Frederick Nightingales'[5] with families to support. They stated that in view of the continuing shortage of nurses it did not make sense to train staff only to lose them to industry or to other countries. In Orpington, for instance, there were 'as many trained nurses in Orpington's factories as in Orpington hospitals'.[6] This problem also existed in other areas, particularly in South Wales and the North of England. In addition, numerous cases were cited of nurses leaving their profession to take up secretarial work since hours of work and levels of responsibility were more favourable in this employment field.

According to some parliamentary members, the answer to these nursing problems lay in a form of coercion. Nurses were trained within the NHS at great expense, they argued, therefore these same nurses should not be allowed to leave and obtain more lucrative positions elsewhere. Others believed that nursing problems could be resolved by encouraging more British rather than foreign girls into the profession. A misguided Labour member for Greenwich claimed that:

> We see many coloured student nurses, but we seldom see a coloured sister, because a coloured sister can go back to her own country and get a good job. Over 5,000 people in this country are in industrial nursing. Industry finds no difficulty in getting qualified nurses, because it outbids the National Health Service. [7]

There was some truth in the claim that industry could outbid the NHS in terms of pay and conditions, but the references to coloured nurses were not based on fact. There were very few coloured sisters simply because most immigrants had been directed into enrolled nurse training. Since enrolled nurses could not be promoted to sister, there were very few coloured sisters working in British hospitals. Immigrant nurses also discovered that enrolled nurse status was not recognised in many countries. Consequently, many immigrants were unable to obtain a good job on returning to their own country. However, this statement regarding coloured nurses was one of many that highlighted parliamentary ignorance regarding nursing problems. Certainly, ministers were not at all sure of nurses' working conditions, holidays and pensions and, for most, the essential point of the debate centred on a moral principle. Should the government be allowed to offer nurses 2.5% simply because nurses would not take strike action to further their claim? As a Labour member pointed out:

> No honourable member had suggested that the social contribution of these people is anything other than first rate. No honourable member on either side of the house would suggest that the rates of pay are reasonable. Only one argument can be put to justify the present situation. That is that the government can get away with it. That in itself is appalling. [8]

There was also considerable criticism of the Whitley negotiating machinery. The Councils were clearly failing to operate efficiently and effectively since most pay disputes were settled by arbitration rather than by Council negotiation. Moreover, the concept of the Whitley Council as an independent negotiating body was called into question. The pay claims of almoners and psychiatric social workers, for instance, were submitted nearly two months before the introduction of the pay pause and an increase of 8% was agreed and approved by the Treasury until the Minister of Health intervened in Whitley negotiations and declared that no offer would be forthcoming. The dispute therefore became the subject of arbitration. Similarly, on 9th January 1962 the Minister of Health attended the management side of the Nurses and Midwives Whitley Council to inform them that nurses would only be offered 2.5%. Since this was a figure that applied to all healthcare professionals, there was no indication that any pay claim was to be assessed on its individual merits.

Meanwhile, teachers and police had threatened militant action and been awarded increases while doctors had forced a Royal Commission into pay and conditions by threatening similar action. The refusal of general nurses to take strike action or even to consider a 'work to rule' served to increase their dependency on public support for pay claims. Radical action was pursued in mental nursing, particularly by members of COHSE, but members of the RCN adhered to the 'no strike rule' (rule 12 of the constitution) in order to define and govern nurse behaviour. As Hart observed, placing the needs of the service before the needs of individual nurses was enshrined in RCN policy and 'clearly, hidden within the prevailing philosophy was the expectation that disobedience would always be followed by punishment'.[9]The policy also allowed that nurses could retain their dignity by adopting the moral high ground and, after much deliberation, nurses were eventually awarded an interim pay increase of an all-round 7.5% which effectively destroyed the 'pay pause'. This interim increase was followed by an award through the industrial court which covered key grades, but was still a far cry from the original claim of 49%. The increases through the industrial court ranged from £2 a year for student psychiatric nurses to £234 a year for senior matrons. This was a pay strategy similar to that meted out earlier to teachers, whereby substantial amounts were awarded to senior staff and new entrants were hardly aware of any increase. In fact, many student nurses and auxiliaries were actually worse off after the award since board and lodging charges were increased. RCN members on the Whitley Council staff side had condoned the refusal to give larger increases to student nurses, claiming that a nurse in training should be regarded as a student. They also claimed that the overall pay settlement was a victory which had been achieved with dignity. COHSE members disagreed and announced in their journal that:

... this view is not shared by students is plain to everybody but the RCN and the Ministry. We leave it to the second year student in charge of a ward on night duty to reflect on the dignity of a gross salary of £345. [10]

The award was particularly cruel since student nurses represented the main body of the nursing workforce and were regarded as students in name only. The Secretary of the Killearn branch of COHSE summed up the plight of the student nurse in a parody of Kipling's poem 'If':

If you can keep your head when all about you are calling for pans and bottles just from you.

If you can hold your tongue when sister shouts to you and make allowances for her shouting too.

If you can make beds and not be tired from the making and being chased round from morn till night.

If you can keep a smile though your feet are aching and yet still think your choice of job is right.

If you can dream and still listen to your tutors.

If you can play and not make life a game.

If you can mix with surgeons, doctors, suitors and treat all these diversions just the same.

If you can bear to hear the one you've tended torn by pain and gasping just for breath.

Or watch and hold her hand till life is ended and pray that she will find her peace in death.

If you can make one heap of all your wages and try to budget till next month's due and fail, and start again on some fresh pages and make it last the four weeks through.

If you can force your knife through bone and sinew and make a meal from some old bullock meatand then get up with nothing in you except the bit you've forced yourself to eat.

If you can treat all sorts of wounds and dressings.

Yet sympathise and keep the tender touch,

and in all this you find God's many blessings and all your patients count but none too much.

If you can work each unforgiving minute and stand each day's long demanding whirl.

Yours is the hospital and everything in it and what is more you'll be a nurse my girl. [11]

Albeit a hollow victory for the nursing profession, the pay award was nonetheless a major defeat for the government. At a time when hospital budgets were frozen and government officials were attempting to curb public expenditure, the increase to nurses had delivered a severe blow to the 'pay pause'. This blow was compounded by the fact that the Minister of Health had unveiled plans to build between 200 and 300 new hospitals by 1973. The implementation of these plans required somewhere in the region of £700 million and the government believed that savings could be made by increasing efficiency levels elsewhere in the service, particularly within the realms of hospital administration. As Treasury officials had acknowledged:

> *... economies in nursing costs were not easy to achieve because individual matrons all had different ideas on the standards required and matrons as a group tended not to have much interest in nursing administration.* [12]

Treasury officials also admitted that the mental health field could not operate without student nurses, but they refused to believe that Britain was experiencing an overall shortage of nurses. Estimates submitted by matrons suggested that 50,000 nursing vacancies existed, whereas the Ministry of Labour suggested 26,000 vacancies. In the absence of accurate information, the Treasury adopted the view that 'the problem was not so much a shortage of nurses but maldistribution of them' and that a more comprehensive analysis of nursing shortages 'might reveal cases of over staffing'.[13]

Since the Treasury considered that nursing shortages were caused by distribution problems rather than problems associated with the recruitment and retention of staff, salary increases were not aimed at improving the lot of the student nurse and the Treasury referred to student nurse pay as a 'training grant'. Clearly, student status was used to excuse the poor pay awards to student nurses. Thus the Treasury terminology had suggested that the government at least paid lip service to the concept of student status. The nursing position was also clear, RCN representatives on the Whitley Council staff side were not overly concerned with raising pay scales for all nursing grades. An analysis of salary negotiations between 1961 and 1963 suggests that the primary focus for RCN members centred on the protection of professional interests. The outcome of negotiations reflected this focus, although status issues were also an important concern. As the staff side rather pompously declared in November 1962:

Whilst they disliked linking the enrolled nurse with the auxiliary the two grades had in common the fact that they were grades without any promotion prospect. [14]

The linking together of these grades for salary purposes had detrimental effects for the enrolled nurse. Since the psychiatric field did not include the enrolled nurse grade, they were paid at the same rate as assistant nurses. (See Table 8.2 for the 1962 salary structure for various nursing grades.) Meanwhile, COHSE members on the staff side of Whitley negotiations had attempted to hold out for improved pay for lower nursing grades, but were far outweighed numerically by RCN members. Various anomalies continued with respect to special duty payments. Ward orderlies continued to be paid overtime rates, for instance, while nurses received an extra £1 per week special duty payment when on night duty. The overriding attitude displayed by registered nurses towards student nurses and ancillary staff was one of superiority.

The AHM had also argued against salary increases for student nurses. According to many matrons, substantial increases to student nurses would undermine the true test of vocational spirit, that of self-sacrifice. One matron proclaimed that 'if a nurse comes to me and shows the slightest interest in salary I have no interest in having that nurse in my hospital, because a nurse must, of course, be absolutely dedicated'.[15] For many student nurses, however, concern over working conditions had taken precedence over salary considerations. Once hospital budgets were frozen, the working hours of orderlies were reduced and students were expected to cover the gaps. Consequently, the time that was normally allocated for meal breaks was reduced and nurses were required to work split shifts. As one student nurse remarked, 'it got so that I would leave home at 7am and return at 9.30pm too tired to do anything but sleep. The Nightingale spirit may be strong but the flesh is weak'.[16] This particular nurse had worked on a ward of thirty patients staffed by one sister, one staff nurse, three students and two auxiliaries. In total, seven staff members were expected to cover a twenty-four hour period. Similar staff-to-patient ratios were to be found on wards throughout the country.

Not surprisingly, standards of patient care deteriorated and nurses failed to express their concerns for fear of victimisation. This situation continued for years in both the general and mental nursing sectors. The problem was first exposed in the mental sector by the Ely Hospital Report, which highlighted cases of patient abuse and revealed the victimisation of nurses. As a direct result of the Ely enquiry, Richard Crossman, Secretary of State for Social Services in 1969, established a Hospital Advisory Service. The service was designed to

Table 8.2
Hospital nursing and midwifery staff, review of salary structure, 1962

Grade	Circular 94 (01.12.1960) £	Award (01.04.1962) £	M/S proposals £	Notes
Student general nurse	299 315 336	321 339 361		No further improvement in training allowances. No change in proficiency allowances for students and pupils
Student psychiatric nurse	352 368 389 452 473 494	378 396 418 486 508 531		No further improvement.
Pupil midwife	305 315 336 404 420 441	328 339 361 434 452 474		No further improvement in training allowances. No proficiency allowances.
Nursing auxiliary[a]	299 315 336 420-525 21(5)	321 339 361 452-564 22(3), 23(3)		No further improvement.
Nursing assistant[a]	352 368 389 452-578 21(6)	378 396 418 486-621 22(3), 23(3)		No further improvement.
Enrolled nurse[a]	452-578 21(6)	486-621 22(3), 23(3)	496-621 25(5)	Minimum further increased by £10. Increments improved and scale shortened.
Staff nurse (general)[a]	525-656 21(5), 26(1)	564-705 22(2), 23(3), 28(1)	575-715 25(2), 30(3)	Minimum further increased by £11, maximum by £10. Increments improved and scale shortened.
Staff nurse (psychiatric)[a]	578-709 21(5), 26(1)	621-762 22(2), 23(3), 28(1)	625-765 25(2), 30(3)	Mental 'lead' £50. Increments improved and scale shortened.
Staff midwife[a]	557-688 21(5), 26(1)	599-740 22(2), 23(3), 28(1)	605-745 25(2), 30(3)	Midwifery 'lead' £30. Increments improved and scale shortened.
Ward sister (general)	656-840 26(5), 27(2)	705-903 28(5), 29(2)	730x30(7)-940, then after 5 years to 1000	Minimum further increased by £25. Maximum further increased by £37 (normal) and £97 (ultimate). Increments improved.

Note: [a] These grades would be eligible for the proposed Special Duty Payments.

Source: RCNA, RCN/13/8/3.

allow nurses and other healthcare professionals to express their concerns over aspects of patient care without the fear of victimisation. The director of the service reported to the Secretary of State and concentrated initially on long-stay hospitals.

Clearly, the Ely scandal had shocked government officials. As Crossman revealed during a conference of the AHM:

> *One of the things that most disturbed me about the Ely Report was the revelation that two nurses lost their jobs because they tried to point out what was wrong. We simply must create conditions where this cannot happen.*[17]

Then, in a more guarded statement, Crossman criticised the attitudes of senior staff towards their juniors, claiming that these attitudes served to perpetuate fears of victimisation. Crossman also expected the Salmon administrative reforms to resolve this problem and stated that, 'It will, if properly introduced, change attitudes of mind so that no nurse should feel inhibited from raising any question affecting patient care'.[18] Crossman's speech, however, was wasted on the matrons. Although they were suitably appalled by the Ely revelations, matrons in general nursing assumed that patient abuse was confined to the fields of mental and mental handicap nursing. The Salmon reforms were also a disappointment and failed to live up to Crossman's expectations. As demonstrated in Chapter 3, the reforms were badly implemented and only served to reinforce existing attitudes.

If attitudes within the AHM had not changed dramatically by 1969, elsewhere in nursing they had. Within the RCN, educationalists had gained ground and policy direction shifted more positively towards improving conditions for the student nurse. The RCN also assumed a more radical approach when dealing with pay disputes. But it would be wrong to assume that these changes were brought about by the traditional RCN membership. Instead, they were the result of a policy decision taken in 1960, the year in which the RCN belatedly opened its doors to men. Thereafter, it was men who successfully turned the tide in nursing and the reasons for this were twofold. Firstly, there were more male nurses working in nurse education, and concerns regarding the student nurse featured strongly in the male political agenda.[19] Secondly, they were more aggressive in pursuing pay since many of them had families to support. Both these changes in policy direction effectively shattered the traditional mould of nursing.

Eventually, educationalists within the RCN were granted an independent review of nurse education, the results of which were published in the Briggs Report of 1972. The Briggs recommendations suggested that nurse training should be more specifically geared towards patient needs. Subsequently, they were used as a basis for the contemporary 'Project 2000' nurse training. In terms of labour relations, the RCN still protected 'professional interests' and adhered to the no strike rule,[20] but they were nonetheless prepared to take some radical action in support of pay claims. The RCN had also developed an uneasy but somewhat fruitful working relationship with healthcare unions. It was therefore a far more unified nursing profession which confronted the government's Prices and Incomes Policy from 1969 onwards.

Never Mind the Ceiling, Nurses Will Raise the Roof!

Between 1963 and 1967 there was a lull in terms of nursing pay disputes, mainly because nurses had agreed in 1965 not to raise any major issue with the Whitley Council for a period of two years. Industrial disputes continued to take place in other employment fields and a total of 2,350 stoppages occurred in 1968, the highest number since 1965.[21] A Prices and Incomes Board was established to ensure that wage increases were maintained in line with productivity but, aside from operating as a restrictive economic policy, the Prices and Incomes Board was largely responsible for the rapid growth in trade union membership within the health service. Since the war, national negotiating machinery had undermined local trade unionists within the health service, but in 1966 the introduction of incentive bonus schemes for ancillary workers in the health service enabled trade unionists at a local level to take part once more in productive bargaining, a process which served to encourage union membership and establish greater bargaining power. This phase of 'new unionism' emerged coincidentally with the formation of district hospitals and an accompanying managerial structure based on private industry.

The proposed new nursing role within the managerial structure of district hospitals prompted a new round of nursing pay claims. Salary increases, according to the RCN, were necessary in order to provide salaries comparable to other occupations and to establish adequate salaries for the new Salmon nursing officer grades, including an appropriate 'ceiling' for the overall structure. Nursing claims, therefore, were submitted to the Prices and Incomes Board in 1967 and duly considered. Nurses suggested a pay ceiling of £4,000 but when the Prices and Incomes Board published its report (no. 60) a pay ceiling of just under £3,000 was advocated. The RCN response was immediate - if this figure was to be the ceiling then nurses would raise the roof.

Significantly, for the first time nurses were comparing their pay rates and responsibilities with those of managerial positions in industry. In previous years the police force had provided a salary indicator, now nurses were expected to adopt management roles and, not unreasonably, expected to be paid management rates. RCN officials sought independent advice from the industrial field before deciding that an appropriate salary for the post of CNO should be somewhere in the region of £4,500 per annum, in view of the fact that a CNO would control a staff of between 1,000 and 1,500. Furthermore, they argued that a low salary ceiling would depress the whole Salmon structure and make it impossible for the nursing profession to attract and retain people of a suitably high calibre to fill top-level positions. For its part, the Prices and Incomes Board refused to budge from its original estimate. The RCN was therefore forced to take action. The 'Raise the Roof' pay campaign which was launched in 1969 became the most prolonged and high profile of any nurse pay claim, and was described by the national press as the 'most vocal and united in nursing history, planned with military precision'.[22]

That the 'Raise the Roof' campaign was organised with military precision was no coincidence. The campaign was organised by an ex-military man, the RCN's Public Relations Officer, Colonel Douglas de Cent, and included specific plans for achieving pay objectives. Nurses were told both to educate their MPs regarding nursing issues and to inform the public of their cause. Special branch meetings were called and recruitment drives initiated. In addition, nurses sought the support of other professional bodies such as the Royal College of Physicians and healthcare unions such as COHSE and NUPE. A high-profile poster campaign was formulated which included the distribution of leaflets and car stickers (examples of posters included in the following pages). Nurses were also given a list of prepared questions with which to confront their MPs, such as: 'What do you regard as a reasonable working week for a nurse?' 'What plans do you have for reducing the overcrowding of wards?' 'Do you agree that there is a need for a national occupational health service? If not, why not?'[23] RCN members were told to stress the two main objectives of the campaign, that of promoting nurse education and raising the roof of the nurse salary structure. As Catherine Hall, General Secretary of the RCN declared, the government should not be left in any doubt that 'nurses are at war'.[24]

Nurses may have been at war, but their real battle was with the Treasury rather than with individual government administrations, since the Treasury remained committed to a policy of wage restraint regardless of changes in administration. As Dr Baly recalled, the process of lobbying MPs revealed that 'there were bastards on both sides of the House of Commons'.[25] A temporary truce between government and nursing camps was achieved in 1970 with the introduction of a one-year 'no strings' pay agreement. Essentially, the agreement provided a 'stopgap' situation while the Whitley Council proceeded to assess the criteria for gradings within the Salmon structure (pay scales shown in Tables 8.3-8.6); though yet again the student nurse was penalised as board and lodging charges were increased, although this action was justified by Crossman on the grounds that, to leave lodging charges unaltered 'would have the effect of reversing the policy of encouraging nurses to live out'.[26]

The one-year agreement was no substitute for a full-scale review of nursing pay, nor did the award achieve an appropriate ceiling for CNO posts. Before taking further action, however, nurses waited for the Whitley Council to assess the

Table 8.3 Pay scales in general hospitals, 1966

Grade	Present scales (£)	New scales (£)
Under age 25[a]		
Student nurse	1st year 395 (+£48 meal allowance) = 443	Age 18 - 525
	2nd year 450 (") = 498	Age 19 - 588
	3rd year 480 (") = 528	Age 20 - 624
Aged 25 and over[b]		
Student nurse	1st year - 565	1st year - 714
	2nd year - 592	2nd year - 744
	3rd year - 619	3rd year - 774
Nursing auxiliary (adult)	565-700	681-846
Enrolled nurse	680-825	801-969
Staff nurse	785-985	930-1182
Ward sister	970-1315	1200-1554
Chief Nursing Officer grade 10(c)	No	2550-3105
Chief Nursing Officer grade 10(b)	negotiable	2814-3414
Chief Nursing Officer grade 10(a)	scales	3102-3702

Notes:

[a] Under the present agreement the rates shown are applicable to the 1st, 2nd and 3rd years of training respectively for all student nurses under age 25 on entry.

[b] Under the present agreement the rates shown are applicable only to student nurses aged 25 and over on entry. The offer proposes 'adult' rates at age 21.

Source: Salmon Report (1966).

Table 8.4 Pay scales in psychiatric hospitals, 1966

Grade	Present scales (£)	New scales (£)
Student nurse	Age 18 495 (+48 meal allowance) = 543	Age 18 - 624
	Age 19 550(") = 598	Age 19 - 687
	Age 20 580 (") = 628	Age 20 - 723
	Age 21+ 1st year - 665	1st year - 813
	2nd year - 692	2nd year - 843
	3rd year - 719	3rd year - 873
Nursing assistant (adult)	665-800	780-945
Enrolled nurse	780-925	900-1068
Staff nurse	885-1085	1029-1281
Ward sister	1070-1415	1299-1653
Chief Nursing Officer grade 10(c)	No	2550-3105
Chief Nursing Officer grade 10(b)	negotiable	2814-3414
Chief Nursing Officer grade 10(a)	scales	3102-3702

Source: Salmon Report (1966).

Table 8.5 Pay scales in local authorities, 1966

Grade	Present scales (£)	New scales (£)
District nurse	856-1237	1065-1464
District midwife	970-1281	1200-1524
Health visitors	1003-1346	1245-1599

Source: Salmon Report (1966).

Table 8.6 Revised numbered scales in traditional structure, 1966

Number of scale	Salary scale (£)	Number of scale	Salary scale (£)
101; 101A; 102	1386-1716	7(a)	1572-1902
103; 103A	1440-1770	7(b)	1506-1836
104; 104A	1572-1902	7(c)	1505-1836
105	1656-1986	8(a)	1845-2200
106; 106A	1761-2136	8(b)	1845-2200
107; 107A	1902-2277	8(c)	1743-2118
108; 108A	2139-2544	9(a)	2430-2880
109	2394-2844	9(b)	2160-2610

The scales in the '200' series (applicable to psychiatric hospitals) to be as above increased throughout by £99.
Note: In addition to the improvements resulting from the above scale, some grades will be paid on scales higher than at present; for example, tutors in each grade in all fields will be paid on scales next higher to their present scales.

		Number of scale	Salary scale (£)
		9(c)	2001-2416
		10(a)	3102-3702
		10(b)	2814-3414
		10(c)	2550-3105

Source: Salmon Report (1966).

criteria for Salmon grading. Subsequently, Whitley grading assessments revealed a considerable amount of confusion regarding the nature of line management, both on the management and staff side of the Council. The ensuing debates highlighted developing tensions between military and industrial models of organisation since the staff side were preoccupied with definitions of authority and frequently failed to understand the subtle changes in management levels. Despite the fact that members of the Council had visited hospitals where pilot Salmon schemes were up and running, the confusion which surrounded nursing 'officer roles' continued to dominate Council proceedings.

As the Whitley Council deliberated, it was clear that government ministers were using delaying tactics with regard to nurse pay claims and the implementation of Salmon. This was particularly true of the Heath administration when the Prime Minister personally intervened in negotiations, although it appeared that no minister wanted to confront the Treasury and, as an outcome of the earlier Plowden Report, government departments were pitted against one another in terms of vying for resources. Dame Irene Ward, Vice-President of the RCN, accused the Secretary of State, Keith Joseph, of cowardice for conforming to the Treasury line. Keith Joseph, however, was preoccupied with health service reorganisation and, as a result, was less inclined to focus on nursing problems.

As the 'Raise the Roof' campaign continued, nurses finally achieved their goal when Keith Joseph was succeeded by Barbara Castle as Secretary of State. Castle recalled that:

> *The Royal College of Nursing, never a militant body, sent a deputation to see me. In determined mood, they told me that we might face a mass walkout of nurses from the NHS unless they were given the independent review of their pay for which they had been asking for some time.* [27]

A strong supporter of earlier nurse pay claims, Castle initiated a pay review body headed by Lord Halsbury.[28] RCN members were placated by this move, but COHSE and NUPE, suspecting that the Labour administration might be short-lived, demanded an immediate increase. Some nurses therefore continued with political demonstrations until Lord Halsbury published his report in September 1974. The Halsbury pay award that followed provided an overall increase of 30% for nurses backdated to 23rd May. However, despite the fact that nurses had been comparing their salaries with management scales, during his deliberations on the subject of nurses' pay Halsbury had reverted to the traditional indicator of nurse salaries. It was, clearly, the police force that yet again supplied the guidelines for comparative pay analysis. As Halsbury confirmed, 'I wanted to give a sister in charge of a ward the same pay as an inspector in charge of a police station'.[29] Despite the nursing shift towards industrial management, government officials still associated the nursing profession with other authoritarian occupations.

The 'Raise the Roof' campaign had taken five years to achieve a review of salary structure and accompanying pay increases and was the longest campaign of its kind for nurses. This sustained effort represented a departure from previous pay campaigns in that nurses were prepared to endorse radicalism. Without strike action, RCN members were successful in highlighting their objectives by demonstration marches and by lobbying MPs. As an apolitical professional body, the RCN were viewed as non-threatening in government circles and were able to exert influence at a relatively high level, whereas COHSE and NUPE, motivated by rank and file nurses, were responsible for spearheading industrial action. Clearly, as Hart has argued, the RCN and COHSE became interdependent during this period. The RCN were able to adopt a tough line in negotiations knowing that, if talks deteriorated, unions would step in and exert real pressure on government policy. This process 'allowed the RCN to await the outcome, choose the best front to put on matters and then claim that any victory was won because it negotiated firmly but sensibly'.[30]

However, the nature of both organisations had changed considerably from 1960 onwards. As previously acknowledged, the incentive bonus scheme introduced by the Prices and Incomes Board had swelled the numbers of both COHSE and NUPE. During the 1962 pay campaign, healthcare unions were weak and badly organised, but in 1969 new unionism had strengthened support at all levels. In contrast, the RCN prior to 1960 was not truly representative of the nursing profession. Membership was confined to female registered nurses who viewed themselves as the professional elite. Although men were admitted to the College in 1960, student nurses in 1968 and finally enrolled and pupil nurses in 1970, the exclusion of large sections of professional members prior to 1960 had severely constrained political activity. The gradual decline in RCN elitism was matched by a corresponding upsurge in radicalism. However, essentially the campaigns in 1962 and 1969 were both prompted by a lack of pay differentials between trained and untrained staff. As such, both campaigns can be viewed as an attempt to reassert the status of the registered nurse above other ranks. The 'Raise the Roof' campaign, however, did confront the problems encountered by student nurses. Furthermore, although the nursing obsession with Nightingale had not disappeared by 1969, it had at least dissipated.[31]

Conclusion

From the mid 1960s onwards there was a gradual political shift within nursing circles, a move away from middle-class conservatism. As a Labour spokesman acknowledged in 1962, most nurses 'would never dream of voting Labour. In a daring moment they might think of voting Liberal, but usually they would for respectability's sake vote for the Conservative Party'.[32] However, even 'respectable' nurses eventually became disillusioned with Conservative policy. The tightening of Treasury control and interference in Whitley negotiations resulted in a more general disillusionment. As Hart has argued, 'if the Treasury did not have a seat on the Whitley Council their spirit sat on the shoulder of government officials who did'.[33] Since the Whitley machinery was time-consuming and frequently used as a means of negating nurse pay claims rather than resolving long-standing disputes, nurses sought more radical alternatives. Whitleyism was used by successive government administrations to depress the salaries of healthcare workers, and delaying tactics in respect of pay claims were not confined to Conservative administrations. Nevertheless, the nurse pay increases of 1970 and 1974 were both sanctioned by Labour administrations. This action served to encourage more registered nurses to join the Labour camp, and to some extent therefore the profession had experienced a political shift.

In terms of professional alignment, however, nurses still had more in common with the police force than with any other occupation. The nursing rejection of educational reform in the late 1940s had precluded identification with the teaching profession and, consequently, nurses were effectively locked into an alignment with other authoritarian professions, although from 1969 onwards industrial management concepts competed with the military model of nursing organisation. The nursing profession therefore fell between two stools, lodged between managerialism and militarism and arguably burdened by the negative features of both.

By far the most important change in direction was that experienced in the field of nurse education. The move towards a theoretical rather than practical based nurse training was motivated by long-standing educationalists within the RCN and given added impetus by male nurses. Although nurses overall were not prepared to relinquish the trappings of military authority, they were, at least by 1970, willing to accept a degree of change on the educational front. But the nature of discipline and socialisation within the nursing service and police force indicated that militarism still exerted a powerful influence within both these occupational fields.

SHORTAGES IN HOSPITALS

WARDS CLOSED
NEW ONES UNOPENED

Why? *Lack of Nursing Staff*

In some wards there are up to 130 patients—all to be cared for by three to four nurses per day shift and by perhaps one or two at night.

As a result, nurses are concerned that the standard of care they like to give must suffer. Recruitment of nurses is falling and one of the reasons is the present level of pay. The nursing profession has always been underpaid. It has been exploited for too long.

Did you know that after three years' hard and exacting training the average cash-in-hand of a newly qualified nurse is £6.14.0. a week?

If you feel that Britain's nurses deserve a fair deal, please support the Rcn campaign for better pay and conditions by writing to the Press, talking to your M.P.s, putting up our stickers and posters, arranging protest meetings and by any other law-abiding and legitimate means.

RAISE THE ROOF!
All Nurses Deserve Fair Pay

ROYAL COLLEGE OF NURSING AND NATIONAL COUNCIL OF NURSES OF THE UNITED KINGDOM
Henrietta Place, London WIM OAB Tel. 01- 580-2646

Poster from the "Raise the Roof" campaign.

Endnotes

(1) *The Times*, 29th March 1962. Mr John Mackay, Secretary of State for Scotland, discussing the all-night Commons debate regarding the nurses' pay claims of 1962.

(2) Nurses and Midwives Whitley Council, 11th October 1949. Report by Professor Thomson.

(3) *Parliamentary* Debates, (House of Commons), 5th ser., 656, 27th March 1962, col.1173.

(4) *The Times*, 19th March 1962. Letter from Catherine Hall, General Secretary of RCN.

(5) Parliamentary Debates, (House of Commons) 5th ser., 656, 27th March 1962, col.1294

(6) *Ibid.*, col.1105

(7) *Ibid.*, col.1182

(8) *Parliamentary Debates,*(House of Commons) 5th series., 656, 27th March 1962, col.1179

(9) Hart, *op cit.*, p.112

(10) MRC, MS229/CO/4/1/15. *COHSE Journal*, July/August 1963

(11) MRC, MS229/CO/4/1/15. *COHSE Journal*, November/December 1963

(12) PRO T291/22. Minutes of a meeting of the Sub-committee of the Committee on Control of Public Expenditure, Health Services, 22nd December 1960, p.3

(13) PRO T291/22 XC15435. Memorandum by the Ministry of Health and the Department of Health for Scotland (CPE(SC3)1), p.1

(14) RCNA RCN/13/8/3. Nurses and Midwives Whitley Council, a meeting between the Management side and Negotiating Committee of the Staff side, 13th November 1962, p.2

(15) *Parliamentary Debates* (House of Commons) 5th ser., 27th March 1962, col.1166

(16) MRC *COHSE Journal*, September/October 1963

(17) RCNA RCN/13/B/16/3. Extract of a speech delivered by the Secretary of State to the Association of Hospital Matrons Conference, 25th April 1969, p.1

(18) *Ibid.*, p.2

(19) As demonstrated in Chapter 3, more men were directed into nurse education because of the lack of promotional opportunities in many clinical areas.

(20) The RCN did not become an official trade union until 1977. Nurses voted to abandon rule 12, the no-strike rule, in 1995.

(21) *British Journal of Industrial Relations*, April 1969, p.289

(22) RCNA RCN RCN/2/4. Newspaper collection (*The Observer*)

(23) RCNA RCH/17/2/4. Extract from the Ten Point Plan of Action for the Raise the Roof campaign.

(24) RCNA RCN/17/2/4. Catherine Hall, extract of a speech given to RCN representative body in Harrogate, 23rd October 1969.

(25) M. Baly, interview, 7th November 1995, Dr Baly was the RCN's southwest representative.

(26) *Parliamentary Debates* (House of Commons), 5th ser., 1799 14th April 1970, , col.203

(27) B. Castle, *Fighting All the Way* (1993), p.470

(28) The Lord Halsbury review body was extended to include all professions allied to medicine.

(29) Castle, *op cit.*, p.472

(30) Hart, *op cit.*, p.131

(31) Nurses still kept all-night vigils by Nightingale's statue as part of the 'Raise the Roof' campaign.

(32) *Parliamentary Debates* (House of Commons), 5th ser, 656, 27th March 1962, col.1205

(33) Hart, *op cit.*, p.76

Chapter 9

Obedience versus Initiative:
The Issue of Nurse Discipline

In view of the paramilitary organisation of both the police and nursing services, professional alignment between these groups was not surprising. However, it was the nature of discipline within these occupational fields that isolated them from other professional groups. A rigid system of discipline was imposed on nurses and police which clearly mirrored the disciplinary code of the armed forces by regulating conduct in off-duty hours in much the same way as in working hours. Nurses and police officers were also imbued with a strong sense of duty. As Lord Crook acknowledged in 1948:

> .. *nurses are rather like policemen: the policeman often finds that the time when he thought he was going to be off duty is the time which, for some pressing reason, he has to give up to duty.* [1]

Strict discipline and a sense of duty were considered by senior nurses to form the essential components of a cohesive nursing service. But a series of official reports from 1932 to 1972 claimed that these very components were responsible for high wastage rates amongst student nurses, although in some instances the timing of these reports was crucial in terms of understanding the overall figures. As Dr Baly observed, wastage rates were unusually high during the compilation of the Wood Report because wartime controls had recently been lifted.[2] Since women who had joined nursing to avoid other forms of war work were leaving the profession at this time, overall wastage figures in the Wood Report were distorted.

Nevertheless, official research continued to reveal a strong connection between high wastage rates and nurse discipline, a connection that was firmly disputed by senior members of the profession. Matrons preferred to believe that wastage was due to the poor calibre of recruits rather than to inherent problems with discipline. As most early reports were not statistically accurate and were not carried out in any depth, matrons were able to reject available evidence for some time. The problem was compounded by the fact that wastage rates were given as blanket percentages with no analytical breakdown. Subsequently, it was often difficult to draw firm conclusions as to exact causes of wastage, although many nurses abandoned training to get married and a percentage failed preliminary nursing examinations.

The lack of flexibility within the organisation of nursing services also contributed to high wastage levels. For instance, there was no attempt to transfer students who had failed one nursing course to another that may have been more suited to their abilities. Nurses who had failed the registration course in the preliminary stages could possibly have coped more easily with the enrolled nurse course. Similarly, nurses who were considered unsuited to general nursing could have been directed into the mental nursing sector and vice versa. The lack of co-operation between nursing sectors precluded this interchange of personnel. In addition, wastage problems were compounded by misleading recruitment propaganda, long hours, poor pay and illness.

The issue of nurse discipline, however, exerted an overriding influence on the levels of nurse wastage. This fact was borne out by the sheer volume of correspondence received by Dr Cohen and included in his 1948 Minority report. Nearly twenty-five years later, during his comprehensive review of the nursing services in 1972, Briggs received similar correspondence.

But while the link between high wastage rates and discipline had been proven, the problem appeared to be insoluble. This chapter, therefore, will examine the precise nature of this discipline and explain why a military style system of control was introduced into nursing circles, and why it was perpetuated. There were also some elements of nurse discipline that did not fit the 'military' pattern and were maternal and emotional in nature. Until 1973 only persons aged twenty-one and over were considered to be adults. Prior to this date, matrons viewed student nurses as children and took it upon themselves to impose moral guidance on their 'offspring'. Maternal control was extended to include all nurses regardless of age and was maintained by a process of systematic intimidation. As Dingwall *et al* have argued with regard to nursing practice, even the:

> *... pointless repetition of mindless tasks was important as a system of discipline which could be used to identify and purge dissident elements. It was the weakening of this control which the leadership feared.* [3]

In some instances matrons were more concerned with controlling student nurses than with aspects of patient care, and all nurses were encouraged to view their first responsibility as being to the matron and training school.[4] A nurse's loyalty to her school could be compared with that of a soldier's loyalty to a military regiment. Each training school competed with another in terms of prestige and many matrons refused to employ nurses who had been trained in schools other than their own. However, the process of occupational socialisation which fostered group loyalty frequently overlooked the needs of patients since loyalty to the ward sister took precedence over loyalty to the patient. Over a period of time, the system of nurse discipline failed to adapt to the changing attitudes within society. Subsequently, the lifestyles of young girls and women did not equate with the outdated expectations of matrons and senior nursing staff.

It is also important to recognise that rigid discipline was not confined to nursing circles but extended to include patients and their relatives. Patients were frequently reprimanded for the slightest misdemeanour and were treated in much the same manner as junior nurses; the medical profession appeared to support this form of control. Medical opinion during the 1940s and 1950s endorsed the view that discipline promoted both physical and mental well being. This system of control provided an emotional and physical barrier between patient and physician. As Dingwall *et al* have argued, existing methods of nurse and patient control:

> ... *eventually declined only when new technologies and strategies of discipline were developed, just as National Service, a similar system of control, came to be seen as irrelevant either to the specialist skills of modern warfare or to the ordering of young men.* [5]

The ramifications of disciplinary measures were extensive, and had long term detrimental effects, both on patient care and the professional development of nursing. It is important, therefore, to understand why the Briggs Report of 1972 merely echoed the findings of Wood and Cohen twenty-five years earlier.

The Nature of Nurse Discipline

In his *Essays on the Welfare State*, Titmuss refers to Weber's theory that the 'discipline of the army gave birth to all discipline',[6] which was based on the fact that since militarism emerged before capitalism, the disciplinary codes of the armed forces were able to serve as a model for industry. This theory, however, ignores the fact that parental discipline existed long before the emergence of militarism and that systematic training in self-control and obedience was also prevalent within some religious orders. Military, parental and religious forms of control combine to provide the three main strands of discipline within society but, although these strands of control can be acknowledged, it is difficult to establish their relative importance. This is particularly true in nursing since the profession was founded on a mixture of religious philanthropy, domestic service and military involvement. The three main strands of discipline, therefore, were inextricably linked.

Nevertheless, by the middle of the twentieth century religious influence within nursing had declined considerably. There were still those who entered the profession full of religious conviction, but early morning prayers, once considered an essential part of the daily ward routine, were abandoned. As scientific advances shifted nursing in the direction of technology, religious conviction was viewed by many to be superfluous within modern nursing practice. Military and domestic influences were not so easily dispelled. Nurse participation in two world wars had revitalised military identification and the role of matron still provided the symbol of matriarchal authority, head of the 'domestic' house and mother figure to young student nurses. The disciplinary methods used to control nurses were therefore derived primarily from military and matriarchal codes of behaviour. In some instances there was an overlap, but for the purpose of analysis the two will be examined separately.

Matriarchal Discipline

With the exception of single sex schools and convents, nursing provided the only example of how women were able to use and abuse their authority within a professional environment. Matriarchal power operated on two distinct levels, both of which imitated the domestic framework of the traditional housewife. Firstly, the ward setting was similar to the family - doctors assumed the role of father, the ward sister displayed motherly characteristics while patients were clearly viewed as helpless children. Secondly, matrons and sisters viewed student and pupil nurses as children and exercised their authority accordingly. Communications between each section of the workforce and patients therefore involved complex power relationships that were not always professionally objective in nature.

For instance, female nurses became emotionally attached to their workplace - a problem which had surfaced during the inter-war period since reduced marital prospects from 1918 onwards had served to emphasise the domestic appeal of the hospital. Matrons exerted tyrannical power based largely on the belief that 'mother knows best and cannot be questioned'. In order to protect this myth, matrons bolstered their authority with a network of disciplinary procedures. This process of protecting female authority could also be detected within home environments. As Bourke noted in her study of English housewives, the matriarch had 'the ability to preclude action and forestall debate'.[7] In establishing a specific sphere of authority supported by unquestionable rules and regulations, the matriarch was able to exert total control over the work environment.

The control exerted by matrons nonetheless relied heavily on the Victorian attitudes of separate spheres and gender expectations. Within a restricted environment under certain conditions, the matron could (and did) remain supreme, but the process of social change that followed the Second World War shook the foundations of this matriarchal power. As medical schools opened their doors to women during the war, female doctors now threatened the paternal role in the ward and, consequently, matrons and sisters became uncertain of their traditional authority. The control of student nurses also presented a problem. As a result of the Butler education reforms, new recruits to nursing were better educated and less inclined to believe that 'mother knew best'. Even the relationship between patient and nurse had shifted. With the rapid introduction of healthcare specialists, nursing control over patient care was substantially eroded. The nursing response to these changes was to adopt an entrenched position. This position was greatly assisted by NHS reforms since matrons were excluded from the policy-making process within the NHS, and many were failing to appreciate the significance of certain changes in medical care and management structure.

The power base of matrons was therefore increasingly eroded. In some hospitals, particularly those in rural areas, matrons managed to retain control of radiography departments and linen rooms. However, by the 1960s many matrons were forced to restrict their authority to nurse training schools. This relegation did not deter matrons from acting as though they still ruled the roost and despite rapid changes in medical technology and accompanying demands for new nursing skills, they resisted change at every opportunity. Nowhere was this approach more visible than in the selection procedures for nursing recruits and in the disciplinary measures used to control junior nurses. As Chambers noted in her study of cadet nursing in the 1960s with regard to selection procedures, interviews did not share any common ground and questions were not directed towards objectively determining a girl's suitability for nursing. Instead, matrons based their interview techniques on a set of personal value judgements. As Chambers has argued:

> ... few of the questions girls were asked at interview could be said to be framed on any scientific basis, nor was there any attempt to assess the answers. Matrons say they possess a 'sixth sense' which helps them pick out the right type of girl for a potential nurse. [8]

But the matrons' claims to have an innate ability to choose the right candidates were not borne out by student wastage rates. In reality, they chose girls who were physically fit enough to endure long hours and demanding work and those who they believed would be able to adapt to harsh discipline. When girls abandoned nurse training, they consoled themselves with the fact that the girls lacked both the stamina and character to become a nurse. This attitude underpinned the belief that nursing was a vocation which only the favoured few could endure and discouraged any internal examination of disciplinary practices. Not that such an examination would have proved straightforward. Matrons and ward sisters operated in a subtle manner, adopting emotional and psychological techniques designed to make students feel guilty and ashamed of their actions. The nature of reprimands highlighted the emotional aspects of nurse discipline since most were unrelated to aspects of patient care.

Matrons, like mothers, were also prone to showing favouritism. One matron, for instance, expressed dismay and a sense of betrayal, simply because her efforts to keep a certain nurse away from undesirable work during the war were not appreciated by the nurse concerned. At the cessation of hostilities the junior nurse had left to take up employment in America, blissfully unaware of the bitterness and resentment felt by the matron who had expected loyalty and gratitude from the nurse in the form of continued service in her hospital.[9] It was also clear that the concerns which dominated the thinking of matrons were based on a framework of preconceived ideas and value judgements, as the following selection of comments from a London matron's register demonstrate:

1) *She had good health throughout but her Irish temperament often led one to believe that she was sullen and resentful.*

2) *She had a critical attitude towards discipline and it was felt that her influence on the younger nurses was not always good.*

3) *It was difficult to keep her, as she had a good opinion of her own ability and her manner was aggressive.*

4) *Undoubtedly she had the ability but she lacked real interest in her work, her interest lay in her pleasures.*

5) *She had a most unprepossessing manner and was highly critical of those in authority in her ward.*

6) *She lacked leadership and had a weak character.*

7) *She had an attractive manner and wore her uniform well but was inclined to modern styles of hairdressing most unbecoming under a nurse's cap.*

8) *She was a bad example to the student nurses and did not attempt to keep the rules.*

9) *She was considered unsuitable as a staff nurse because she was caught sunbathing naked on a roof top during off duty hours.*

10) *She was capable, intelligent, well able to rise to responsibility and kind in her dealings with patients but she became very self-assertive and had a critical attitude towards authority. She was personally untidy and unprofessional in her manner and appearance. She was socialistic in her views and made strong endeavours to influence her colleagues in this respect. We were not sorry to lose her services.* [10]

The concerns of matrons and sisters did not appear to shift over time. One nurse working at Southmead Hospital in Bristol during the 1960s stated that, 'most nurses left the profession because of the bitchiness displayed by senior staff towards junior members'. As Ann Uren recalled:

When I could not afford to buy an anatomy book in my first year, I was told by my tutor that I should not be in nursing at all if I could not afford the books. There were two good sisters in the hospital and a charge nurse who was fine, but all the rest were pretty awful. [11]

Senior nurses also acted very much as moral guardians. Accordingly, they demonstrated disapproving attitudes towards certain boyfriends and some sisters were known to change a student nurse's shift without prior notice in an attempt to prevent a romantic liaison.

However, despite the negative and oppressive features of nurse discipline, many believed that it achieved positive effects on overall morale. Recollections from Betty Hall in Cumbria stated that, 'There is no doubt that the strictness and conditions made us a very cohesive group, who supported each other at all times'. [12] Research also indicated that nurses either adapted to or rejected discipline during the first year of their training. Of the nurses who rejected discipline, most objected to the restrictions which governed their private lives rather than those that were included in the normal ward routine.

Nurses understood the need for some rules, even those which governed their personal grooming. For instance, fingernails needed to be kept short to prevent patients from being scratched during nursing procedures and hair needed to be styled so as not to come into contact with a patient's wound or food. These rules were necessary to protect the patient. Young nurses also appreciated that matrons needed to adopt a parental role. The imposition of evening curfews represented part of that role. Rules that were imposed within nurses' homes, however, were petty and unnecessary, They were not allowed to keep vases on windowsills or photographs on dressing tables, many were prevented from taking a bath after ten o'clock in the evening and most were prevented from talking to male staff. In some instances, letters and phone calls were monitored. This intrusion into a nurse's private life formed part of a wider process of social indoctrination that combined features of parental and military discipline.

It can also be argued that nurses desperately needed a form of discipline which was not based purely on the domestic framework of matriarchy in order, firstly, to diffuse the emotional nature of matriarchal control and, secondly, to provide a broader base for exercising authority. Establishing legitimate authority within the hospital environment had presented problems for women since the initial negotiations with administrators, governors and doctors regarding nursing policy. The outcome of these negotiations depended on the value placed on the nursing contribution to medical care. An analysis of medical committee minutes at a variety of hospitals revealed that doctors placed great emphasis on the smart appearance of nurses and viewed them as an essential support to their own medical prestige. But since doctors needed to establish their reputations by curative treatments rather than by 'caring' for patients, they believed that nursing was of limited value in terms of overall medical impact. From the outset, therefore, nursing was a precarious profession. There was no means of measuring the success or failure of nursing care, a problem that was compounded by the fact that nurses could not agree on any common ground regarding nursing tasks and policy formulation. This situation allowed for the proliferation of numerous specialist groups and sub-groups which eroded nursing authority and depressed nurse status. In terms of authority, therefore, nurses needed a clearly defined method of establishing spheres of influence in relation to other healthcare professionals. But instead of developing new models of discipline, nurses reinforced their matriarchal authority with a combination of aristocratic and technocratic militarism.

Military Discipline

As previously acknowledged, military discipline within nursing realms originated with the Nightingale reforms. Nightingale herself was known to have endorsed the concept of strict discipline and was prone to making comparisons between nurses and soldiers. Discipline, she argued, was what made people 'endure to the end'. Training in obedience was essential to make sure that every person 'did their own duty rather than every man going their own way'.[13] Subsequently, aristocratic army traditions and customs were incorporated into nursing - ceremonial presentations of badges and medals, rigid class stratification and, more importantly, the disciplinary procedures that were believed to produce characters of strong moral fibre. Identifying the military features of nurse discipline, however, presents a problem since maternal discipline displayed similar features. It can be argued that military personnel possibly based systems of discipline on their own childhood experiences of punishment. The public humiliation of a soldier in front of his colleagues, for instance, can be likened to a mother punishing one child in front of another to set an example although, as Bowman acknowledged in his study of the history of the Royal College of Nursing:

> *The Army believed that discipline could only be maintained if commissioned officers were kept within a high Brahmin caste and if non-commissioned officers ruled by terrorism. Once a private soldier got his first stripe, therefore, he was required to bully and roar. Precisely the same thing happened with the average nurse on promotion, not because of anything wrong about the dedicated nurse's character but because the hospital tradition of the time, and for a long time afterwards, demanded it.* [14]

Bowman further claims that nurses and soldiers enjoyed exerting military style authority, a statement that explains to some extent why there was little attempt to change the pattern of this authority.

Having incorporated military-style bullying and forms of public humiliation into the professional structure, nurses at a later date endorsed the concept of technocratic military efficiency. This involved, amongst other features, inspections of wards at which nurses stood by their patients' beds like privates on parade, waiting for matron to comment on the state of the ward and their personal appearance. In addition, nurses were required to report on and off duty. They were not required to salute their superiors, but deference to authority was, nonetheless, extreme. One nurse recalled having to 'flatten against the passage walls when matron or sister passed'.[15] In dining areas nurses of differing ranks sat at different tables and were required to stand when a sister or matron appeared in the room. Nurses were also segregated according to rank in nurses' homes and sick bays, within which many juniors were forced to endure verbal abuse and breaches of confidentiality regarding their personal lives. As Salvage has remarked, 'The stories of nurses' inhumanity to nurse are hardly believed when told to friends outside the job, yet are all too familiar inside it'.[16] Evidence suggests, however, that some nurses adapted well to such a lifestyle and accepted the system in a 'military spirit'. As a Manchester nurse declared:

> *I was very obedient and fell into the discipline quite happily*
> *actually, because my father was a soldier in both wars and he was*
> *a very disciplined man, so it didn't worry me too much.* [17]

Others were not so compliant. Most nurses resented not only the petty rules but also the fact that they were confined to hospital 'sick bays' during periods of ill health. The introduction of sick bays indicated a 'motherly concern' for the well being of sick nurses. Medical care was provided within sick bays on much the same basis as that provided in normal hospital wards. Nurses were confined to their beds and treatment administered as required. But sick bays also represented another example of military influence. The compulsory nature of confinement to sick bays reflected a nursing obsession with the issue of malingering. As Cooter and Bourke have pointed out, military officials were preoccupied with this problem and consequently the work of military medical officers resembled that of detectives who attempted to catch the culprits by a variety of means. This preoccupation resulted in numerous cases of misdiagnosis, sometimes with fatal consequences. Many medical officers appeared content to follow military orders regarding potential malingerers, but there were others who found the whole process of trapping malingerers distasteful. Bourke cites the case of a Lancashire medical officer who 'claimed that his colleagues were obsessed with the 'debasing idea' that the men went sick to escape duty' and refused to co-operate in military plans to catch malingerers.[18] Senior nurses had no such compunction in dealing with junior nurses who reported sick. They, like the military officials, were obsessed with the notion that nurses feigned sickness in order to escape duty. Refusing to believe that their juniors were really sick, sisters frequently (and without notice) entered the rooms of student nurses to check the existence of illness for themselves.

Clearly, nurses received unsympathetic treatment with regard to their physical ills and this lack of sympathy was extended to their emotional problems. Despite the stressful and sometimes difficult nature of their work, nurses were presumed to be able to cope with any situation. There were no support networks to assist nurses through difficult periods and nurses who admitted to experiencing emotional trauma in the course of their work were believed to have an underlying character weakness. One newly appointed staff medical officer at the Royal London Hospital in 1967 expressed his concern at the level of emotional disturbance displayed by nurses. The Medical Officer, Dr K.

Brown, consulted his predecessor Dr Bouford with regard to the problem. The latter, however, managed to convince his colleague that when the working conditions of a nurse were taken into consideration, 'the figures were not unduly high'.[19] The problem was perpetuated by senior nurses who believed that juniors should either have the strength of character to withstand emotional trauma or should acknowledge their weakness of character and abandon training. This attitude reinforced the superiority of senior nurses within the professional hierarchy. Seniors deluded themselves into believing that they were tougher than the 'new generation' of nurses. Those who failed to complete their training were viewed as weaklings who lacked stamina and fortitude, whereas the cruel and unnecessary discipline was regarded as an essential component of a Darwinian style selection procedure, an initiation process whereby only the strongest, most dedicated nurses would survive to become part of the elite.

Senior nurses successfully managed to dominate young girls, but this domination did not extend so easily to male and older nurses. The system of discipline relied on girls being recruited at an impressionable age. Matrons and sisters controlled these girls by continual surveillance both in and out of working hours. The behaviour and appearance of these girls was closely monitored and punishment tasks were meted out to anyone daring enough to flout the petty rules and restrictions. Following the Second World War the male influx into nursing challenged this position. Senior nurses were less than comfortable in giving out orders to men since men were more inclined to question these orders and less prepared to endure sarcastic comments with regard to their behaviour and appearance. Older female nurses were also less compliant than their younger colleagues, particularly those who worked on a part-time basis. As the educational levels of recruits improved, discipline became more severe as senior nurses felt increasingly threatened by their own insufficient knowledge base. Internal conflicts arose between nurses of similar status and much of this conflict at ward level centred on the character versus intellect debate. Sister tutors and ward sisters in some areas literally fought over student nurses, with neither group managing to assert their authority in a calm professional manner. The problems centred on the time allotted for nurse education. Ward sisters were reluctant to allow student nurses to attend lectures, claiming that nursing skills were more easily acquired in the ward environment, while tutors insisted that theoretical knowledge was important if nurses were to understand the implications of nursing care. The onus was frequently placed on student nurses to resolve the situation by acting as go-betweens on an indefinite basis. As a Manchester nurse recalled of her training in the 1960s:

> *... the ward sisters and tutors were daggers drawn in an undeclared war. We had to go and tell our ward sister we were due for a lecture, the tutors never did it, they always left it to us to make arrangements on the ward and the ward sisters always seemed to obstruct it ... not quite always, it depended on the personality of the sister, but a lot of them did go out of their way to prevent it. The ward sisters and the sister tutors never seemed to speak.* [20]

This undeclared war on the wards highlighted two major problems within nursing. Firstly, that the character versus intellect debate operated at a very basic level and prevented any real progress in the field of nurse education; and secondly, that senior nurses were unable to assert legitimate authority in areas where the military rank structure did not provide a clear dividing line. In the case of ward sisters and sister tutors, the former took precedence over the latter. The rank structure did not dictate this precedence, but the ideology that underpinned professional behaviour did. As previously acknowledged, a nurse's character was considered to be all-important while educational achievements were undervalued. As a result, sister tutors were always slightly unsure of their position and at times genuinely afraid of being dismissed. Ward sisters were able to capitalise on this insecurity and often refused to allow student nurses to attend classes.

The power struggle between nurses of similar ranks also demonstrated a fundamental distortion of the military model as applied to the civilian nursing profession. Registered nurses during the war had fought for 'officer status' and equated their rank with commissioned officers. As Bowman has pointed out, however, the role that registered nurses adopted vis-a-vis student nurses was that of the non-commissioned officer. The military hierarchy had been adopted by nurses, but without much consideration of the finer details. In theory, ward sisters and tutors occupied the same status position within the nursing hierarchy, but the structure of this hierarchy prevented parity of authority. Prevailing attitudes towards management skills also highlighted differences between military and nursing organisation. The military placed great emphasis on teaching man management, nurses assumed that management techniques would be acquired naturally. Nurses were therefore encumbered by a distorted version of military organisation. More importantly, over a period of time the nursing features which reflected 'aristocratic' and 'technocratic' militarism bore little relation to contemporary military organisation since, in order to attract recruits and adapt to new technology, the military had moved in the direction of education and professionalisation.

Despite this shift in direction, the type of discipline meted out in military circles did not alter dramatically. In addition to the petty rules and bullying, discipline was used to emphasise class distinctions and racial superiority. Viewed in this context, nurse discipline was an exact copy of military discipline. As Chambers argued in her contemporary study of nursing during the 1960s, 'Nowhere, except perhaps in military circles, is discipline so rigid and tradition so fixed as in a hospital'[21] although, regardless of the harsh nature of this discipline, nurses appeared to have their own reasons for perpetuating a military style regime - reasons which were never quite understood by those working outside the profession, and not completely understood by those working within it. These reasons are therefore worthy of further analysis.

Reasons for Discipline

The most consistent operational argument put forward by senior nurses in support of discipline centred on the need to protect patients from the risk of clinical error. Clearly there was some validity in this argument and a few regimented procedures were designed specifically to safeguard patient interests. For instance, prior to surgery, rigorous identity checks were made to ensure the correct patient received the correct treatment. Similarly, nurses protected the personal property of patients with a series of checks and counter-checks. But, with regard to general discipline, it was the parallels drawn between nursing work and the work of military personnel that dictated disciplinary techniques. In both, staff were trained to deal with unexpected situations and consequently, in order to guarantee a synchronised response to clinical emergencies, training ultimately relied on the unquestioning obedience of subordinates. As Dr Baly observed, in nursing, 'like the army, crisis tends to be normal and the operating theatre and the battlefield are notorious for not lending themselves to sweet reason'.[22] Nurses and soldiers were therefore trained to respond to orders rather than to question them.

There was also a time factor involved in disciplinary techniques. Since the ratio of qualified nurses to students was poor, there was little time for senior staff to instruct or supervise juniors adequately. In view of this problem, a system of nursing practice founded on authoritarian rule was considered to be the most efficient method of deploying staff. However, by far the most important reason for strict discipline at ward level stemmed from the need to hide professional insecurity. As Salvage has argued, most senior nurses were ill-prepared to exert authority and felt the need to 'cling to the trappings of titles, uniforms and privileges'.[23] This argument is supported by Baly who states that, 'the process of democracy in nursing was delayed because technical knowledge advanced with such rapidity that each generation was stranded on the beach of insecurity, and insecurity breeds aggression'.[24]

The existence of professional insecurity undoubtedly fostered a reliance on strict discipline, but there was also a distinct shift during the twentieth century towards a more 'masculine' military style of administering care. Nurse discipline reflected this shift. On several occasions, both during and after the Second World War, nurses had been accused of inefficiency. These accusations had emanated primarily from members of the medical profession, although even official nursing reports such as those provided by Wood and Cohen had questioned nurse efficiency. Nurses had responded to these accusations by adhering to the concept of military efficiency. Whereas, in previous years, the profession had maintained an 'angel of mercy' image, from 1939 onwards the 'angel' was replaced by the 'officer'. Status issues came to the fore once more and military style discipline was considered essential in order to promote an efficient image.

Discipline was also used to reinforce the nursing hierarchy. A survey conducted in 1961 by Professor Revans revealed that nursing authority was instrumental in dictating both supervisory attitudes and the stability of the workforce. These attitudes also affected patient care in that hospitals that were unable to retain their nurses recorded longer periods of individual patient stay, whereas the reverse occurred in hospitals where the nursing workforce was stable. Supervisory attitudes played a fundamental role, therefore, in both nurse and patient turnover, attitudes which in many hospitals were clearly out of step with other sections of society. Almost half the sisters interviewed in Revans' study, for instance, believed that:

> *Most young people today have had too soft an upbringing. Education today gives the student nurse too much theory and sisters can devote time to instructing the student nurse only at the expense of what may be more important demands.* [25]

There were also those who believed that the tradition of segregating nurses of differing status at meal times was essential to ward efficiency.

Throughout the survey, ward sisters were asked several questions designed to measure their attitudes towards the supervision of junior nurses. From a sample of three hundred and fifty sisters, fifty per cent were in total agreement with the military style discipline. As Revans observed:

These questions may, no doubt, reflect the popular image of authoritarianism within the hospital or the military tradition into which the nursing profession as it is at present known is often said to have been born. But the responses of the sisters themselves remove any suggestion that these images exist only in the popular imagination; the tradition of hierarchy is an essential part of the nursing ethic. [26]

However, if discipline during working hours served to underpin the nursing hierarchy, disguise professional insecurity and protect patient interests, then discipline in non-working hours served a different purpose. Nurses were expected to behave impeccably at all times because conduct was considered to reflect the status of respective training schools. Therefore, just as an off-duty soldier was expected to behave in ways which would not bring his regiment into disrepute, a nurse was expected to behave in ways which did not bring discredit to her training school. Discipline was also used to create a class elite. Thus, registered nurses in some hospitals were not allowed to associate with ward maids or porters. For example, one:

> ... *staff nurse (mature in years), returning late one night after spending her rest day in London, was seen to stop and converse with the lodge porter for a few minutes. Next day the matron severely censured her, saying that it was unseemly conduct.* [27]

Examples of this kind could be quoted indefinitely. For matrons, however, the rationale behind this type of discipline was simple; training schools were highly competitive and a school's reputation was all-important. Exerting control over nurses during off-duty hours was merely one method of protecting this reputation.

Equally, discipline was viewed as a professional character trait, an essential part of a difficult initiation process. But while some sisters exerted authority in the firm belief that discipline improved a nurse's character, there were others who abused their authority. As Dame Kathleen Raven recalled of her own training, 'Some of the sisters were harridans, some were almost sadistic. They were jealous of the younger nurses and their behaviour could be very petty'.[28] Almost forty years later, hostile communications between senior and junior nurses continued to present a problem. The Briggs Report of 1972 noted that nearly all the complaints concerning the nursing profession related to the behaviour of nurses themselves, 'with stress on the power motivation of nurses, not on their compassion, and with talk not of 'ladies of the lamp' but of 'dictatorial automatons'. 'They're the ones who make hospitals into institutions' was one of the most sweeping comments of 1971'.[29] Clearly, therefore, nurse discipline was perpetuated to some extent simply because nurses enjoyed power.

However, the disciplinary system was not merely designed to control nurses. Patients and visitors were also expected to adhere to rules and regulations. Strict visiting hours kept relatives and friends in abeyance, despite the fact that many nursing tasks could have been performed on the wards by relatives, thus relieving the work of nurses during periods of staff shortages. The emphasis on ward appearance dictated patient behaviour. Many patients were prevented from lying on their beds once they had been made and bedside lockers were supposed to be six inches away from the bed, regardless of the convenience to patients and, in some cases, bedridden patients were prevented from reading newspapers because the print soiled the sheets. There was, however, at least some recognition that not all patients could be subjected to discipline of this nature. Nurses at Great Ormond Street had noted that:

> It will not be found that the same regularity and order can be maintained amongst children as among the adults. Order and discipline there must be, or the child will not be happy, but the ward that is tidied to perfection, in which the little ones look like well drilled soldiers, when the look of liberty is absent and nothing is out of its place, is hardly suggestive of the happy heart of a child. [30]

Specialised hospitals for children, therefore, had subsequently relaxed their disciplinary procedures, although children's wards in general hospitals did not appear to do likewise.

Similarly, patients suffering from mental illness or handicap presented a problem in terms of control. While patient discipline in general hospitals was administered by nurses, patients in mental hospitals were subjected to the rule of the 'drill instructor'. Responsible for the implementation of physical training programmes and the supervision of recreational activities, drill instructors could make a significant contribution to patient welfare. Without appropriate medical training, however, it was difficult for instructors to assess the physical well being of mental patients. Consequently, measuring the patient response, positive or otherwise, to this form of discipline was virtually impossible. As COHSE acknowledged, 'Most of the instructors are ex-service men with a good knowledge of physical training, some having army qualifications. They are not required to have mental nursing qualifications'.[31] Discipline was therefore imposed on patients with no accurate means of determining whether or not 'drill procedures' improved mental health. This was a scenario that highlighted a far wider problem - if patients and nurses were to be continually subjected to discipline, how were the effects of this discipline to be measured?

Effects of Discipline

The adverse effects of discipline on the recruitment and retention of nursing staff were first identified in the Lancet Report of 1932.[32] Subsequently, a series of official reports had claimed that discipline was responsible for high wastage rates amongst student nurses and low patient morale. From the Wood Report of 1947 through to the Briggs Report of 1972, nurse discipline emerged as a significant problem, both in terms of nurse training and clinical practice. However, the problem did not become a major issue in all nursing fields since strict discipline was associated primarily with the hospital environment. As Maclean's contemporary analysis of nursing pointed out, 'away from the strict hierarchy of the hospital, nurses can often exercise a gratifying amount of autonomy. They are in the front line of the organisation, a long way from the military style supervisors who command them'.[33] Community nurses, therefore, and those working in the public health field, were in a position which favoured the use of personal initiative. Their work was largely unsupervised and patients were evaluated within the family and work setting. Consequently, the nurse-patient relationship evolved as one of co-operation rather than domination. Each community nurse worked independently and clinical decisions were made without recourse to the directives of senior staff.

In contrast, divorced from family surroundings, the hospital patient was dominated by nursing staff. The nurse-patient relationship was depersonalised at every level and patients were expected to adopt a 'stiff upper lip' attitude towards their pain and distress. Nurses were encouraged to refer to patients by their medical condition and orders such as 'wheel over the male collapse', or 'bring in the acute female now'[34] were not designed to inspire patient confidence. In addition, nursing staff erected a barrier of secrecy between patients and medical knowledge while the complexities of medical diagnosis and treatment were shrouded in equally complex terminology. Rare disclosure of information, therefore, only served to increase patient anxiety. Nevertheless, hospital nurses were expected to 'cultivate a deliberate detachment in the interests of efficiency'[35] and were reprimanded for expressing open concern. As a result, patient anxiety was not always alleviated and recovery was frequently delayed.

Several studies suggested a link between nurse discipline and delayed patient recovery, but this link was not conclusive since, in terms of patient welfare, it was impossible to separate discipline from other aspects of treatment.[36] By the same token, there was no evidence to indicate that discipline made any positive contribution to patient care. As a COHSE official admitted with regard to mental patients, 'In the early stages all physical training is largely achieved by imitation and in many cases the patient never gets beyond this stage'.[37] Clearly, disciplined training programmes for the mentally ill were of dubious value, as were the rules and regulations that governed general patients. It was, however, difficult to prove that strict discipline was detrimental to patient care.

Establishing a link between discipline and nurse wastage was also problematic. According to official reports the nature of nurse discipline remained the most significant cause of nurse wastage. Since, however, various other factors influenced wastage rates, the effect of discipline on these rates was not easily evaluated, particularly as the link was somewhat obscured by confusing statistical data. Ministry of Health figures differed from those of the Ministry of Labour, which differed yet again from those issued by the General Nursing Council. Figures published in the COHSE Journal also frequently conflicted with official estimates. Furthermore, as Levine had pointed out in his analysis of hospital personnel, wastage rates were easily distorted.[38] A seventy per cent wastage rate, for example, could merely reflect a seventy per cent job turnover once a year or, alternatively, a thirty-five per cent turnover of jobs twice a year. Measurements of wastage, therefore, needed to take account of normal turnover rates, as distinct from staff instability. Statistical analysis of nurse wastage throughout this period, however, failed to produce figures other than in the format of crude turnover.[39] Nevertheless, despite the discrepancies in available figures, all reports concerned with nurse wastage acknowledged two main facts: firstly, that the highest degree of wastage occurred during the first year of training and, secondly, that the nature of nurse discipline influenced wastage rates throughout training.[40]

The problem of high wastage rates was not confined to nursing circles. When considering an age range of between twenty and twenty-five years, an average wastage rate of twenty-four per cent was recorded for women in both the teaching and nursing professions. Clearly, this correlation reflected the most usual age for women to marry and have children. Wastage rates amongst policewomen also followed this general trend, but more nurses began their training at a much younger age than did recruits to other professions. In the case of cadet schemes, nurse recruits were only sixteen and many abandoned training during the first few months. As Moores pointed out in his 1971 analysis of the problem, patterns of nurse wastage were more comparable with the industrial employment sector than with other professional groups. A study conducted in Lancashire, for instance, revealed that nurse wastage was little different from the wastage problems experienced in a local appliance factory. A straightforward comparison in this context was not particularly illuminating, however,[41] as it would be reasonable to assume that recruits to the nursing profession entered training with slightly more commitment to their chosen employment field than those embarking on factory work. Furthermore, the tendency for all employees to leave their jobs appeared to decrease as their length of service increased.

Comparisons between the mental and general nursing sectors were more helpful in identifying actual causes of wastage than were comparisons with other employment areas. Studies revealed that the mental nursing sector experienced a far higher dropout rate than the general nursing sector and that mental nurses were far more likely to leave the profession for reasons other than discipline-related problems. The mental nursing field was dominated by men and recruits tended to be much older than recruits to general nursing. Many men entered mental nurse training as a second career option, having previously failed to succeed in other employment fields. As the majority of these men had families to support, wastage levels were largely determined by pay issues.

Other issues that influenced wastage rates in this sector included the geographical isolation of mental hospitals and the risk of violence since, despite advances in drug therapy, it was not uncommon for mental patients to launch violent attacks on nursing staff. In some regions the dropout rate for recruits continually exceeded 70 per cent, a problem exacerbated by the low status afforded to mental nurses within the profession as a whole. Clearly, these problems encountered by mental nurses were different from those experienced by their colleagues working in the field of general nursing. In terms of finding solutions, however, nurses were no nearer to resolving these problems in 1969 than they had been in 1939. MacGuire's research into wastage revealed a connection between the educational levels of recruits and their ability to complete training, which supported the view that wastage levels could only be reduced once the calibre of nurse intake was improved.[42] Hospital matrons endorsed this view.

But in 1964 this view was challenged in a study conducted by Revans, which argued that wastage levels were also determined by an 'institutional effect'. According to Revans, the ability of recruits to complete their course frequently depended on the morale of individual hospitals and the quality of their training schools. Aspects of discipline, training programmes and inter-personal communications were all responsible for creating the 'institutional effect' which, in turn, influenced staff morale. Thus, certain institutions were able to produce good results with poor quality recruits, while others produced poor results with good quality recruits. Revans' study was highly significant in that it highlighted problems associated with nurse discipline that had hitherto been ignored. As Moores acknowledged in his 1971 study:

> *Even now many matrons still feel the only solution to the wastage problem is through an upgrading of the calibre of intake. This is perhaps explained by the fact that to admit that, in their hospital, matters could be improved by better planning, better communications, etc. is a bitter pill to have to swallow.* [43]

Refusal to acknowledge substantial failings in the areas of nurse management, supervision and training could be detected in the prevailing attitudes towards new recruits. Senior nurses had assumed that strict discipline was essential to the moulding of a nurse's character. In their view, high wastage rates were the result of girls 'being too soft' and lacking in character. Consequently, the 'institutional effect' on nurse wastage was severely underestimated.

It was not surprising, therefore, that since the profession had overlooked the obvious effects of discipline on patient morale and nurse wastage, the more insidious effects of discipline on professional development were also ignored. Systematic training in obedience had stifled nurse initiative. Just as mental patients imitating the drill instructor had failed to get beyond the stage of constant repetition, so junior nurses imitating their seniors had also failed to escape repetition. This was a problem fostered by the distortion of the military nursing model within the civilian hospital environment. Medical military personnel had recognised that most recruits consisted of two distinct personality types - those who preferred to have decisions made for them and those who wanted to take part in the decision-making process. Military officials, therefore, had concluded that the armed forces needed to cater for both personality types. Some recruits, they argued, were capable of producing independent ideas within contemporary society, but initiative and self-reliance in others was stultified by the 'all-providing welfare state'. [44]

As senior military personnel acknowledged, in terms of professional advancement it was important to direct and encourage the 'thinking personality', while simultaneously providing an adequate environment for the characters who were 'content to have everything decided and done for them'. [45] Herein lay the crux of the problem for civilian nurses for, although the military nursing model had catered for both types of individual, civilian nursing had failed to cater for the 'thinking personality'. In the process of adapting the military nursing model for use in the civilian field, an essential component of this model had been lost. Without this component civilian nurses were clearly unable to direct professional development. As the Briggs Report of 1972 pointed out, there was 'considerable evidence from nurses in training about petty restrictions and authoritarian systems of control' and student nurses were 'treated as initiates who have to be moulded into the system rather than as free agents who might make useful suggestions about how it could be changed'.[46] Discipline within the training school environment was therefore largely responsible for professional stagnation.

Just as the effects of discipline on nurse wastage rates were not easily evaluated, neither could the role of discipline in professional development be measured with any degree of accuracy. Nor could it be argued that the concept of professionalism as interpreted by nurses necessarily improved patient care, since professionalism in nursing did not challenge the existing system of organisation. Instead, professionalism was used to justify the practice of withholding formal training from a large body of nursing personnel. As Salvage has argued, professionalism in nursing 'assumes that relatively few nurses should be highly trained and supervise larger numbers of untrained people; it does not even consider the idea of spreading education more widely to give a basic training to more people'.[47] Professional aspirations had centred on the need to protect the interests of registered nurses within the overall nursing hierarchy, rather than with the pursuance of policies which would benefit patient care. Naturally, since strict discipline underpinned the hierarchy, registered nurses were reluctant to relinquish this feature of 'professional' organisation.

Nevertheless, while the majority of nurses appeared to be in favour of authoritarianism, it would be wrong to assume that there were no dissenting voices amongst the nursing population. Whereas most nurses were prepared to accept discipline in the ward environment, they were less inclined to accept restrictions that caused infringements in their personal lives. Such infringements were responsible for an important, and frequently overlooked, consequence of nurse discipline, namely the growth in the unionisation of nurses. Doris Westmacott, nurse leader within COHSE, for instance, 'became involved in unions as a ward sister because she had become irritated by rigid regulations regarding permission to go out in the evening'.[48]

As Table 9.1 reveals, other nurses took similar action (these figures do not include members of the National Union of Public Employees).

Table 9.1 Membership figures: COHSE and RCN, selected years, 1947-77

Year	COHSE	RCN
1947	40,000	—
1950	—	*44,239*
1967	66,240	47,366
1973	*113,401*	*92,773*
1977	200,455	95,668

Source: C. Hart, Behind the Mask (1994), p.133.

In addition to giving impetus to the unionisation of nurses, discipline also prompted the government-initiated policy of encouraging nurses to 'live out'. This was a policy strongly resisted by the General Nursing Council and hospital matrons. Eventually, a compromise situation was reached whereby student nurses were required to be resident in nursing homes for the first year of their training and allowed to be non-resident from the second year onwards. Even then, many hospitals did not adopt this policy until the late 1960s, which was a time when Ministry of Health officials were producing numerous circulars demanding the relaxation of restrictions imposed on nurses in 'off duty' hours - circulars which had little impact on the infrastructure of nurse discipline. The shift away from such discipline only began once the educationalists within nursing became dominant. The Briggs Report of 1972 was the result of long-standing pressure from nurse educationalists and signalled a change in direction for nurse organisation. Status issues were, for the first time, associated with educational achievement. Subsequently, military identification was no longer considered the only frame of reference for maintaining nurse status. From this point on, the military style discipline which had given nurses their sense of power and reinforced their 'officer class' status began to subside.

Conclusion

The origins of military-style discipline within civilian nursing were located in the Nightingale reforms of the nineteenth century. After the Nightingale system had ossified, it can be argued that the perpetuation of such authoritarianism was unavoidable since the organisational framework of this system left little room for experimentation in management techniques. There were attempts to identify and resolve discipline-related problems but, viewed within an 'institutional' context, it was difficult to separate discipline from the overall hospital infrastructure. Despite government efforts to moderate nurse discipline, therefore, patient care and nurse training continued to suffer from the adverse effects of authoritarian rule. Change became possible only when the profession ceased to view military identification as the primary reference point for nurse status.

The decline of nurse discipline coincided not only with a shift towards theoretical nurse training, but also with the general demilitarisation of society. The demise of National Service, the emergence of anti-military propaganda generated by the Vietnam War, and the more 'liberal' generation of the 1960s, had combined to undermine the respectability of military values. Nevertheless, military style discipline was not totally eradicated from civilian nursing circles. As Salvage's contemporary account of nursing reveals, senior nurses in 1985 were still obsessed with the prospect of nurses malingering to escape their duty. Interfering with nurses' private lives was still considered to be a 'normal' function of sisters and matrons, while severe criticism of a nurse's personal appearance and conduct both on and off duty remained a feature of the nursing environment.[49] The pervasiveness of nurse discipline was not surprising given the rigidity of the organisational system but, as Salvage argues, 'The vigour with which many nurses express their hostility - including senior nurses themselves remembering their own experiences as juniors - suggests some deeper malaise beyond the normal pattern'.[50]

It can be argued that this malaise was specifically associated with female authority. The ways in which women exerted their power over other women suggested a degree of competitiveness and jealousy in the work setting that was never openly acknowledged. Nurses had accepted that the male dominated medical profession was in some way responsible for suppressing nursing aspirations, but they were less inclined to put their own house in order. As a predominantly female profession, nurses had clearly failed to support other females. Rather, they had stifled the initiative of young girls and blocked the career paths of older women by denying them access to flexible hours and childcare facilities. In other words, nurses suffered the effects of intense matriarchal oppression in the workplace, an oppression which was far greater than any exerted by the patriarchal medical profession. Furthermore, while it is impossible to separate the military and maternal elements of nurse discipline, it is evident that senior nurses firmly believed such discipline to be an essential component of nursing professionalism.

As Clay has argued:

> *In the deepest possible irony, nurses who kick up a fuss, lose their temper, or fight for patients' rights in an overt way, are labelled deviant, stupid, politically extreme or - especially - unprofessional. Only nursing could find itself equating professionalism with acquiescence, subservience, silence and obedience.* [51]

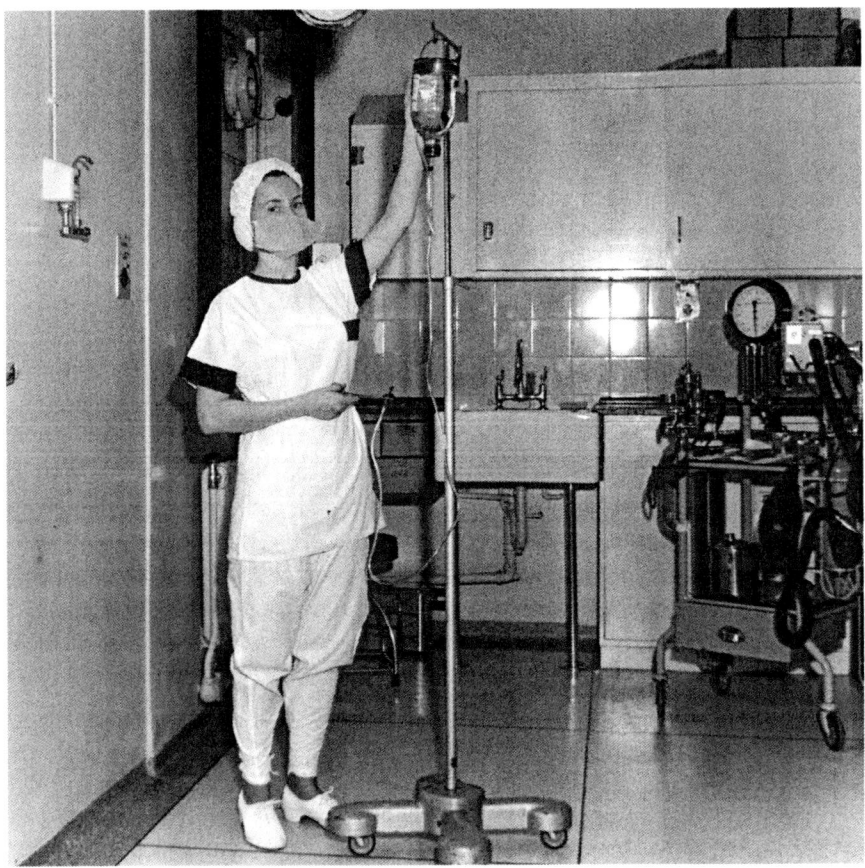

May 1963 - Cardiff Royal Infirmary. Trousers are introduced for nurses working in operating theatres. Trousers were introduced for hygiene reasons rather than comfort. The picture shows Sister Prosser, who designed the new uniform.

Endnotes

(1) *Parliamentary Debates* (House of Lords), Official Reports, 1159, 9th November 1948, col.300
(2) M. Baly, *Nursing and Social Change* (1980)
(3) R. Dingwall, A. Rafferty and C. Webster, *A Social Introduction to Nursing* (1988), p.118
(4) U. Maclean, *Nursing in Contemporary Society* (1974), p.66
(5) Dingwall *et al, op cit.*, p.118
(6) R. Titmuss, *Essays on the Welfare State* (1958), p.85
(7) J. Bourke, 'Housewifery in working class England, 1860-1914', *Past and Present*, 143 (1994), p.182
(8) V. Chambers, 'Cadet Schemes and their Impact on the Recruitment and Wastage of Nurses', unpublished Ph.D. dissertation, University of Manchester (1960), p.206
(9) This account was recorded in 1946 by Miss Clare Alexander, Matron of the Royal London Hospital, and can be found in the Matron's register of that year.
(10) The Royal London Hospital Archives, *random extracts from matrons' registers 1940-1950*. The nurses referred to in the seventh, eighth and final quotations, respectively, left voluntarily, the former two to take up secretarial work and the latter to become an industrial nurse.
(11) A. Uren, Oral History Interview conducted 1st August 1995
(12) B. Hall, letter to author, 10th May 1994
(13) M. Baly, *As Miss Nightingale Said* (1991), p.91
(14) G. Bowman, *The Lamp and the Book, story of the Royal College of Nursing* (1967), p.105
(15) N. Houghes, 'One hundred years of training at Great Ormond Street, 1878-1978'. *Great Ormond Street Nurses' League Journal*, (1978), p.18
(16) J. Salvage, *The Politics of Nursing* (1985), p.82
(17) Wellcome Unit for the History of Medicine, Manchester tape N19. N. Hawthorne, oral history transcript, p.6
(18) J. Bourke, *Dismembering the Male* (1996), p.93. See also R. Cooter, 'Malingering in Modernity: Psychological Scripts and Adversarial Encounters During the First World War', in R. Cooter, M. Harrison and S. Sturdy, eds., *War, Medicine and Modernity* (Stroud, 1998), p.125-48
(19) Royal London Hospital Archives: Nursing Advisory Minutes, 1968
(20) Hawthorne, *op cit.*
(21) Chambers, *op cit.*, p.199
(22) M. Baly, *Nursing and Social Change*, p.230
(23) Salvage, *op cit.*, p.81
(24) Baly, *op cit.*, p.230
(25) R. Revans, *Measurement of Supervisory Attitudes* (Manchester, 1961), p.2
(26) *Ibid.*, p.12
(27) MRC MS229/6/C/HA/3/1/15. W. Hayden, 'Nurse Wastage'. This example was one of many quoted by Will Hayden, Secretary of Guildford Hospital Branch of the National Union of Public Employees.
(28) Dame Kathleen Raven began her training at St Bartholomews Hospital, London, in 1933.
(29) A. Briggs, *The Briggs Committee Report on Nursing* (1972), p.28
(30) N. Houghes, 'A hundred years' training at Great Ormond Street'. *Nurses League Journal*, p.6, 1978
(31) RCNA RCN/13/B/16/1. Letter from Assistant General Secretary, COHSE, to Frances Goodall, 30th May 1951.
(32) The Lancet Commission of Inquiry into the Nursing Services, 1932
(33) U. Maclean, *Nursing in Contemporary Society* (1974), p.142
(34) *Ibid.*, p.117

(35) *Ibid.*. p.127

(36) The most notable of these studies was undertaken by Professor Revans for the Nuffield Provincial Hospitals Trust in 1964, entitled *Standards for Morale Cause and Effect in Hospital.*

(37) Letter from the Assistant General Secretary of COHSE to Miss F. Goodall, *op cit.*

(38) E. Levine and S. Wright, *Analysing Turnover among Hospital Personnel* (1957), p.37-42

(39) The Ministry of Health conducted surveys of hospital wastage in 1967 but results were not revealed.

(40) GNC figures for nurses leaving training in the first year were 34% in 1957 and 41.5% in 1959.

(41) B. Moores, 'Patterns of nurse wastage'. *International Nursing Studies,* 8 (1971), p.63

(42) J. Macguire, *Threshold to Nursing* (1969)

(43) Moores, *op cit.,* p.62

(44) Wellcome Institute for the History of Medicine Archives, London RAMC/1976/9/1. Royal Army Medical Corps, *Field Training School Precis Gen 6 - Man Management,* p.5

(45) *Ibid.*

(46) Briggs, *op cit.,* para.229

(47) Salvage, *op cit.,* p.100

(48) MRC MSS/229/6/C/CO/7/20D. Westmacott, oral history interview conducted 25th April 1979

(49) Salvage, *op cit.*

(50) *Ibid.,* p.82

(51) T. Clay, *Nurses Power and Politics* (1987) p.46

Chapter 10

Conclusion

This study of British nursing history between 1939 and 1969 has revealed a series of missed opportunities in terms of nurse organisation and professional development. There were, however, fundamental problems inherent within the overall framework of healthcare delivery. Despite an obvious need for a more coherent approach towards health education, for instance, successive government administrations refused to make any substantial financial commitment to the field of preventative medicine. Moreover, intense political lobbying by members of the medical profession largely dictated government policy in this respect. Doctors relied on 'curative' rather than 'preventative' treatments in order to establish their individual reputations and subsequently used their political leverage to persuade ministers that funds should be concentrated within the hospital environment.

The framework for providing civilian healthcare was therefore, in itself, a distortion of military healthcare delivery. The civilian was ignored by the NHS until his or her illness or injury required attention. In much the same way, the soldier was expected to be healthy until he was injured on the battlefield. However, within the military environment there was a greater emphasis on health education and, since most soldiers were expected to be fit at all times in preparation for combat, the military approach to preventative medicine differed dramatically from the civilian approach. While the soldier was expected to be fit for battle, the civilian was not necessarily expected to be fit for industry.

If the overall framework for healthcare delivery was less than ideal and governed for the most part by senior members of the medical profession, then nurses needed to make a concerted effort in order to effect change. Clearly, however, many nurses did not want change and the profession's overriding concern with status served to overshadow all other issues, including those that surrounded aspects of patient care. It can be argued that, in view of the bitter struggle for professional recognition, concern with nurse status was justified, but this concern became an obsession that dictated nursing policy. The militarisation of the profession during the second world war did have the effect of elevating nurse status in the short term. Ironically, however, by providing an immovable obstacle to reform, this same militarisation policy ultimately undermined nurse status in the long term. Civilian nurses interpreted military 'officer' status in terms of social class and failed to appreciate that the primary function of an officer was to provide leadership. Consequently, civilian nurses identified with 'officer' status without fulfilling the officer role. While the Horder Reports of the 1940s acknowledged that officer class nurses were urgently required to provide professional leadership, nurses evidently did not share this sense of urgency.

The Horder Reports were received favourably by the profession, primarily because they were commissioned by the RCN and merely reflected current nursing opinion. Horder had therefore predictably endorsed the military hierarchy and stressed the 'officer' status of registered nurses. In contrast, the government-initiated Wood Report had advocated a more egalitarian system of nurse training which was rejected by senior members of the RCN and GNC. This move was equally predictable and, in many respects, the profession's reaction to Horder and Wood epitomised the overall nursing stance throughout the 1950s and beyond. Subsequently, the militarisation of nursing escalated during the post-war period. While the military model of nursing became increasingly anachronistic within a rapidly changing society, military influence within nursing did not begin to decline until the late 1960s. Even then, this shift in direction was primarily due to the decision by the RCN to welcome male nurses into their ranks, since the proliferation of male RCN members from 1960 onwards gave considerable impetus to the movement for educational reform.

In terms of the relationship between government policy and the nursing profession, however, a shift in direction could be detected by the late 1950s. Government plans for the large district hospital system of the 1960s exposed the need for nurse administrators. Ministers therefore began to concentrate on the administrative structure of nursing rather than on mere recruitment figures, although the long-awaited Salmon administrative reforms did little to change the military structure of nursing. As Walby and Greenwell have noted, the reforms succeeded in 'exacerbating the internal hierarchy within nursing and benefiting male rather than female nurses'.[1] Nevertheless, this statement is misleading in that within the pilot schemes, where Salmon was implemented as intended, the new administrative system provided an efficient managerial structure for nurse organisation. In the majority of hospitals, however, Salmon was implemented in an ad hoc fashion and nurses assumed new titles without undergoing vital management training.

The Salmon system benefited male rather than female nurses, but this outcome was not the result of a pre-planned conspiracy against female nurses. In fact, the Salmon system favoured males because it favoured those who were in positions within nurse education, and there were more males working within nurse education simply because female nurses had denied them promotional opportunities within clinical areas. It can also be argued that since female nurses had failed to provide support networks for their colleagues with children, any system of nurse organisation would inevitably favour male nurses.

Salmon did succeed in drawing attention to the existing military model of nursing since the administrative reforms represented the first real challenge to the traditional nineteenth century nursing structure. Without the widespread introduction of management courses for nurses, however, the 'corporate' challenge to the military model was destined to fail. Nurses simply used the Salmon system to reinforce officer status and strengthen the professional hierarchy. Neither can it be argued that the nursing analogy with the military entirely dissipated, as demonstrated by the following quote from a hospital consultant recorded in Walby and Greenwell's contemporary study of medicine and the nursing professions:

> *A ward sister runs the place in the doctor's absence and she is like*
> *the sergeant major who then gives the next tier, like the nurses, the*
> *orders of what needs to be done. So if you clash with the sister,*
> *that's a problem, there's a complete obstruction in the middle*
> *between the commander and the troops.* [2]

Racism, social injustice and the ongoing 'character versus intellect' debate within nursing circles is also indicative of the military legacy. Albeit inconsistent with the rejection of reform, attempts to reintroduce the minimum educational level formed the basis of GNC policy during the post-war years. At the same time, the GNC failed to recognise that this isolated policy was not enough. The educational content of nurse training needed to be substantially increased in order to attract more highly educated recruits once this minimum level was re-established. Attempts to combat the military legacy of institutional racism and social injustice within the nursing framework have significantly failed, as a recent study conducted by Aliyar Darr at Bradford University discovered. Student comments such as 'Oh it's the Pakis not turning in' or 'it's the Pakis coming in late, it's the Pakis this and the Pakis that' were being left unchallenged by lecturing staff. [3]

However, perhaps the greatest irony in British nursing history originated with the relationship between Florence Nightingale and the nursing profession. Nurses worshipped Nightingale as their heroine and created a myth that was supported by a seemingly limitless amount of Nightingale iconography. But while nurses were busy trying to attract the 'right' type of middle-class girls into the profession, and associating their registered status with that of military officer class ladies, Nightingale had actually stated that working-class girls made better nurses. Nightingale had acknowledged that 'ladies' would inevitably become the hospital matrons, but only because they were educated, not because they were 'ladies'.

She also voiced considerable doubts regarding the 'despotic power' of matrons.[4] In April 1878 Nightingale wrote that:

> *My views are exceedingly altered as to the supremacy of the matron. It did very well for me whose fault is subserviency and civility. It does ill for matrons whose fault is the love of power and lawlessness towards medical and other authorities and for matronships where there is not a strong and intelligent administration with power and duties running parallel to the matrons.* [5]

Again in May 1887, Nightingale voiced doubts with regard to matriarchal authority:

> *I am not so sure now that nursing should be so entirely in the matron's hands, now we [the Nightingale Fund] have no dominance over her. We have recommended people lately who ought not to be within a mile of the hospital.* [6]

In view of the subsequent problems associated with nurse discipline and student wastage rates, Nightingale's doubts were well founded. Clearly the military structure of nursing served to foster the abuse of power, but it also highlighted the oppression of women by other women, the existence of which has been frequently overlooked by feminist historians. In addition to acting as an obstacle to reform, therefore, military influence within nursing provided women with an opportunity to exert power within a traditional 'male authority structure'. In an effort to gain status, nurses had continually identified with the military and masculinity but, in the long term, status could not be sustained by this process. As the leading protagonist of nurse militarisation, Dame Katherine Jones had noted in 1944 that, 'Status cannot be created or justified by such [military] scaffolding alone'.[7] Nearly thirty years later the British nursing profession had discovered the validity of this statement.

Endnotes

(1)   S. Walby and J. Greenwell, *Medicine and Nursing Professions in a Changing Health Service* (1994), p.67

(2)   *Ibid.,* p.19

(3)   E. Leach, *The Times Higher,* 'Racism Rife in Nursing' 5th March 1999

(4)   M. Baly, *Florence Nightingale and the Nursing Legacy* (1986), p.181

(5)   *Ibid.*

(6)   *Ibid.*

(7)   PRO WO/222/178. Dame Katherine Jones, 2nd September 1944

Bibliography

Unpublished Sources

Theses and papers

Baly, M. (1995) *Nursing Logistics as a Legacy of War*. Unpublished conference paper given at the RCN 'Legacy of War' Conference, Cavendish Square, London, 31st May.

Chambers, V. (1960) Cadet schemes and their impact on the recruitment and wastage of nurses. Unpublished thesis, Manchester University.

Markham, J. (1995) *From Service to Civilian Practice*. Unpublished conference paper given at RCN 'Legacy of War' Conference, Cavendish Square, London, 31st May.

Pyke, D. (1996) *The Work of Guttman in relation to Paraplegic Patients*. Seminar paper given at the Wellcome Unit for the History of Medicine, Oxford, 1st March.

Archives

Aldershot Museum

The Queen Alexandra's Royal Army Nursing Corps Military Museum, Aldershot. Diaries of individual QA nurses, 1939-46.

Public Record Office material

Ministry of Health files MH55-80

Treasury T161-291

General Nursing Council:
    DT41/39-46, 57-58, 60-85
    DT48/GNC minutes on microfilm
    DT16/307-309
    DT16/156, 633, 591, 585, 548, 547, 322, 333, 532, 484, 348, 349
    DT34/68, 89-128
    DT5-47

Ministry of Labour: LAB8-33

Board of Trade: BT31/23218/143404

War Office: WO/106-222

Airforce: Air20-49

Admiralty: ADM1 series 1 codes 1-20, 56-1, 56-2, 56-3, 56-4, 56-9, 56-10, 56-11

Royal College of Nursing Archives

British Commonwealth Nurse War Memorial Fund: minutes of council (RCN 1/)

Industrial disputes: (RCN 13/33/2-15/1/18)

Insurance and legal: (RCN 13/ED/1-/3)

International Council of Nurses: Congress Reports, study tours and overseas nurses (RCN 12/1-18)

Labour Relations, pensions and pay: (RCN 13/EA/3-13/EC/15)

Oral history transcripts:

Dame Elizabeth Cockayne: RCN T/10

Dame Kathleen Raven: RCN 13/ED/1

Royal College of Nursing, Cavendish Square, London: RCN film collection, *Handmaidens and Battleaxes* (1987), Australian Broadcasting Company

Press and PR: (RCN 17/2/1-RCN 17/4/45)

Speech by Enoch Powell to RCN Conference, (1963) RCN 29

Files and committee papers: (RCN 20-31) (RCN 12/4/2-/3) (RCN 12/5/1-2)

Labour Relations Department: (RCN 13/A/7/ 13/D/1) (RCN 17/8/1-26/5/)

Recruitment: (RCN 26/37/1-26/1/46). Includes reports of the RCN Reconstruction Committee (Chairman Lord Horder), London, RCN 1942-49

Nursing Times Advisory Board, Minutes and editors' reports, 1958-1963: RCN 7/3

Ad hoc Committee on role of health visitors: RCN 7/3

Course committees, programmes, correspondence and administration: (RCN 7/4-19)

Correspondence with Department of Health, Ministry of Health, 1945-1978: (RCN/7/10)

Modern Records Centre, Warwick

Annual Conference papers: MS/229/CO/4/1/12

Confederation of Health Service Employees files: MSS/229/16/HA/3/1/15; MSS/ 299/6/C/HA/3/1/1 to /27

Confederation of Health Service Employees journals: MS/229/CO/4/1/15

Oral history tapes:

Doris Westmacott: MS/229/O/C/CO/7/20

Iris Brook: MS/229/6/C/CO/7/1

Wellcome Unit Records

The Wellcome Unit for the History of Medicine, Manchester: oral history transcripts obtained from senior nurses working in the Manchester area during the 1960s: tapes N1-20.

The Wellcome Unit for the History of Medicine, London: Royal Army Medical Corps Records 1939-1976

Hospital Archives

Bristol Records Centre, Bristol Royal Infirmary:

Nursing minutes 1939 to 1950

Great Ormond Street Hospital Archives:

Nursing minutes 1938 to 1968

Medical minutes 1938 to 1968

Hospital League Review 1939 to 1963

Radcliffe Royal Infirmary: nursing advisory minutes, 1939 to 1966, plus minutes of Nursing Services Sub-committee of 1948 to 1966, Banbury and District Management Committee.

The Royal London Hospital Archives:

Matrons Registers 1938 to 1958

Nursing Advisory minutes 1939 to 1969

Medical minutes 1948 to 1969

Nurses Hospital League review 1939 to 1945

Nurse recruitment statistics 1939 to 1969

The Warneford Hospital Archives, Oxford include material from the Radcliffe Royal Infirmary and Banbury and District Management Committee

Lambeth Palace Archives

Language papers 164 and 172; Fisher papers 10-18; 1957, 190 and 224-6; 1951, 90.

Imperial War Museum, London

Royal Army Medical Corps: 116.326, K51271. Story of RAMC

516.326, E7314, G. Anderton. Journal RAMC, vol.9, no.2

516.326 and 516.81, E159900. RAMC and RADC Army Nursing, Gale and Polden, Aldershot

616.326 Acc K61363. Sponsored units of RAMC, TAVR, 1967-69

516.326, E14797. KSLI and Herefordshire LI Regimental Journal, vol.16, no.92

516.326, E7314. J.C. Barnetson, Journal RAMC, vol.XCVI, no.2

516.326, 14941. R.E. Barnsley, Overlord, 1944, 85th magazine, no.50

316.326, K48899. Various typescripts, army medical arrangements

516.326. Life in our hands, MacGibson and Kee: maps, papers and diagrams

516, E7314. Journal, vol.XCVI, no.4

516.326, 47884. Airborne medical services

516.326, HMSO 31809. Cabinet office papers

516.326, 49677

516.326, E7314. Journal RAMC, vol.LXXXVIII, no.1

516.326, E7314. Journal RAMC, vol.XCIII, no.4

516.326, K13549

516.326, E7314. Journal, vol.LXXXVIII, no.2 and 3

516.326. Journal, vol.100. TA and medical services, G.M. Frizelle

316.326, E7341. Journal, vol.XCIV

516.326, E7341. Journal RAMC, vol.IXXVII

516, K65098. Journal, vol.LXIII, no.228

116.326, 65541

166.326, K52775. RAMC History Museum

116.326, K48745

516.326, E17660

516.326, 27688. BTA weekly journal.

516.326, E7314. Journal, vol.XCII, no.5

516.326, HMSO 57794. Medical services in war

K37217. Medical women's federation

516.326, E7314. RAMC, vol.XCVI

516.326, K8021. GHQP notes on military hospital administration

616.326. Ministry of Defence papers

HMSO, standing orders for QAS incorporating amendments 1-16, 50039.

Ministry of Information, K11179

616.325. Journal, vol.105, no.4

516.326, E14550. Army Nursing Services Gazette, vol.XIV and XV

516.326. United services and empire review, vol.LXXXIII, no.4305-4307

War Office, HMSO 42954

HMSO 38736, 616.326

516.326, E7314. Journal, vol.XCL, no.3

K37744, Westminster Hospital in war

41 UK 3, Cabinet Office, HMSO, 31809

531, Ministry of Health, 26961

531, K52481

531.1. War Office, tables and graphs, HMSO, 24467

631.1. Ministry of Defence, naval, HMSO, 57818

45 UK 721, Cabinet Office, HMSO tables and graphs (civilian)

536.172, K6834. Central Emergency Committee for Nursing Profession, 1939. Civil Nursing Reserve

536.172, K16402. Hospital Matrons Association

536.172. Utility Nurse, Chaterson, p.VII and 101

536.172. GNC 1940, K16178

536.172. GNC 1939, K16179: proposed changes in training and examination of nurses due to wartime conditions

536.172, K16180. Extracts of minutes, November 1944

536.172. GNC war years 1939-1945, K16228

17428. Picture Post, 22nd November 1941

536.172, K8143. HMSO Civil Nursing Reserve

536.172, K9540, K8142, K8616. Ministry of Health

536.172, K12070. Ministry of Information reference division, health nursing midwifery services

Ministry of Labour, 1944, employment of women: how orders affect nurses. PL146/1944, K10823

536.172, HMSO, K9547, K9798, K9354

536.172, K9775. Recruitment and distribution of nurses, guidance manual for hospital authorities, 1943

HRL 4, HMSO, K9491, 1943

HMSO, K12304

536.172, HMSO K9584. Report of VAD Committee, tables and plans

536.172, K16728. Queens Institute of District Nursing, 1939-1945

536.172, K16093, 1949. War activities of midwives

536.172. Sector Matrons Committee, 1939-1947, minutes and reports, two folders

536.172, 557.1, 29929. Hospital nurses, 1941

Oral history interviews

Baly, M. RCN representative for the south-west during the 'Raise the Roof' campaign: interviewed in November 1995

Gruber von Arni, Colonel E.E, RRC/QARANC, Director of Education, Queen Alexandra's Royal Army Nursing Corps: interviewed in October 1993

Salmon, B. CBE. Chairman of the 1966 Salmon Committee: interviewed in October 1993 and June 1994

Titley, J. Matron in Chief of the Army, Navy and Air Force Nursing Services (retired 1995): interviewed in October 1993

Uren, A. student nurse at Southmead Hospital, Bristol, 1960-1963: interviewed August 1995

Official Publications

Command Papers

1938 Report of the Scottish Departmental Committee on Nursing. Cd. 5866

1944 White Paper, The National Health Service. Cd. 6502

1946 Report of the Committee on the Provision for Social and Economic Research. Cd. 6868

1946 Report of the Ministry of Health for the Year Ended 31st March Cd. 7119

1946 Report of the Royal Commission on Equal Pay. Cd. 6937

1948 Cotgrove, S. Technical Education and Social Change: first annual report of the Advisory Council on scientific policy. Cd 7465

1954 Ministry of Health Statistical Report on the Nursing Workforce. Cd. 9566

1972 Briggs, A. The Report of the Committee on Nursing. Cd. 5115

Other official publications

1932 Report of the Lancet Commission on Nursing

1939-1973 Parliamentary Debates (House of Commons)

1939-1950 Parliamentary Debates (House of Lords)

1939 The Athlone Interim Report conducted by the Rt Hon the Earl of Athlone appointed by the Ministry of Health in Co-operation with the Board of Education. HMSO

1942-1949 Nursing Reconstruction Committee chaired by Lord Horder, GCVO, MD published in the RCN Annual Reports of 1942, 1943 and 1949. In 1942: section one, the assistant nurse; in 1943: sections two and three, education, training and recruitment; and in 1949: section four, the social and economic conditions of the nurse.

1943 Wartime Social Survey into the Recruitment of Nurses conducted by Box. K, and Croft-White. E, HMSO

1943 Reports of the Nurses Salaries Committee conducted by Lord Rushcliffe for the Ministry of Labour and National Service in Co-operation with the Department of Health for Scotland. HMSO

1947 The Working Party into the Recruitment and Wastage of Nurses conducted by Wood, R. HMSO

1947 Report of the Expert Committee on the Work of Psychologists and Psychiatrists in the Services. HMSO

1948 The Minority Report on the Recruitment and Training of Nurses conducted by Cohen, Dr J. HMSO

1948-1973 Reports and Minutes of the Whitley Council for Nurses and Midwives

1953 The Work of Nurses in Hospital Wards survey conducted by Nuffield Provincial Hospitals Trust

1960 The Measurement of Supervisory Attitudes in the Nursing Profession, conducted by Revans, Professor R. for Manchester Statistical Society

1964 The Standards for Morale in Hospitals, Cause and Effect, conducted by Revans, Professor R. for the Nuffield Provincial Hospitals Trust

1966 Report on the Structure of Senior Nursing Staff conducted by Salmon, B. HMSO

1967 The Recruitment of People with Higher Educational Qualifications into the Police Service. HMSO

Journals and Newspapers

The British Journal of Industrial Relations, 1960 to 1970

The British Medical Journal, 1948 to 1970

The Journal of British Nursing, 1939 to 1955

The Bulletin and Scottish Pictorial, 1940 to 1955

The Daily Telegraph, 1949 to 1950

The International History of Nursing Journal, 1995

Ministry of Labour Gazette, May 1947.The Survey of Manpower Trends in Great Britain 1946-1951

The Lancet, 1945 to 1960

The Liverpool Daily Post, 1949 to 1951

Nursing Illustrated, 1939 to 1943

The Nursing Mirror, 1960 to 1970

The Nursing Times, 1955 to 1970

The Royal United Services Journals, 1950 to 1970

The Times, 1950 to 1972

The Woman Teacher, 1945 to 1950

Secondary Sources

Books

Abbott, P. and Sapsford, R. (1987) *Women and Social Class*

Abel-Smith, B. (1960) *A History of the Nursing Profession*

Baly, M. (1980) *Nursing and Social Change*

Baly, M. (1986) *Florence Nightingale and the Nursing Legacy*

Bannister, R.C. (1979) *Social Darwinism, Science and Myth in Anglo-American Thought*. Philadelphia

Baskett, I.F.W. (1991) *The Amateur Military Tradition 1558-1945*. Manchester

Bassett, J. (1992) *Guns and Brooches*. Australia

Bell, G. (ed) (1967) *Organisations and Human Behaviour*. New Jersey

Benn, T. (1987) *Out of the Wilderness: Diaries 1963-1967*

Bidwell, S. (1977) *The Women's Royal Army Corps*

Berghann, V.R. (1981) *Militarism, History of an International Debate*

Blenkinsop, D. & Nelson, E.G. (1972) *Changing the System: a study of organisational change in a hospital nursing service*

Bourke, J. (1996) *Dismembering the Male*

Bowman, G. (1967) *The Lamp and the Book: a history of the Royal College of Nursing*

Bridges, D. (1967) *A History of the International Council of Nurses 1899-1964: the first sixty-five years*. Philadelphia

Broadley, M. (1995) *Patients and People*

Brogden, M. (1982) *The Police Autonomy and Consent*

Brown, R.G.S. & Stones, R.W.H. (1973) *The Male Nurse*. London: G. Bell & Sons

Cambray, P. & Briggs, G. (1947) *The Official History of the Humanitarian Services of the War Organisation of the British Red Cross Society and the Order of St John of Jerusalem 1939-1947*

Carpenter, M. (1977) The new managerialism and professionalism in nursing. In: Stacey, M. (ed), *Healthcare and the Division of Labour*

Castle, B. (1990) *The Castle Diaries 1964-1970*

Castle, B. (1993) *Fighting All the Way*

Chapkis, W. (ed) (1981) *Loaded Questions, Women in the Military*. Amsterdam

Clay, T. (1987) *Nurses, Power and Politics*

Cooter, R. (1993) Medicine and War. In: Bynum, W.F. & Porter, R. (eds), *Companion Encyclopaedia of the History of Medicine*

Cotterell, A. (1943) *Royal Army Medical Corps*

Critchley, T.A. (1967) *A History of the Police in England and Wales 900-1966*. Letchworth

Crossman, R. (1979) *The Crossman Diaries*, ed. Howard, A.

Davis, F. (ed) (1966) *The Nursing Profession*. Five sociological essays which form part of a group of publications on organisations and professions prepared in conjunction with the Centre for Social Organizational Studies at Chicago University under the direction of Morris Janowitz. New York

Dingwall, R., Rafferty, A. & Webster, C. (1988) *A Social Introduction to Nursing*

Doyal, L. (1980) *Migrant Workers in the National Health Service: report of a preliminary survey prepared for SSRC by the Department of Sociology*. Polytechnic of North London

Encel, S. (1968) *Armed Forces and Society*. Netherlands

Enloe, C. (1980) *Ethnic Soldiers*. Athens

Enloe, C. (1993) *The Morning After: sexual politics in the Cold War*

Fielding, N.G. (1988) *Joining Forces: police training, socialisation and occupational competence*

Forsythe, W.J. (1983) *A System of Discipline 1819-1863*. Exeter

George, V. & Wilding, P. (1972) *Social Values and Social Class*

Giddens, A. & Hall, D. (1982) *Classes, Power and Conflict: classical and contemporary debate*

Glaser, W.A. (1970) *Social Settings and Medical Organisation: a cross-national study of the hospital*. New York

Godber, G.E. (1976) *The British National Health Service*. United States Department of Health and Welfare: NIH 77 1205

Granshaw, L. & Porter, R. (1989) *The Hospital in History*

Hart, C. (1993) *Behind the Mask*

BIBLIOGRAPHY

Hooper, C. (2,000) Manly States: Masculinities, International Relations & Gender Politics.

Howard, D.L. (1960) *The English Prisons*

Howes, R. & Stephenson, M. (1993) *Women and the Use of Military Force*

Howlett (1995) *Fighting with the Figures*. Central Statistical Office, HMSO

Jacobs, J.B. (1985) *Socio-Legal Foundations of Civil-Military Relations*. New Brunswick

Janowitz, M. (ed) (1981) *Civil-Military Relations: regional perspectives*

Klein, R. (1983) *The Politics of the National Health Service*

Levine & Wright (1957) *Analysing Turnover among Hospital Personnel*

Lovell, J.P. & Kronenberg, P.S. (1974) *New Civil-Military Relations*. New Brunswick

McBryde, B. (1989) *Quiet Heroines*. Herts

Macdonald, D. (1995) *The Sociology of the Professions*

Macguire, J. (1969) *Threshold to Nursing*

Maclean, U. (1974) *Nursing in Contemporary Society*

MacNaulty, A.S. (ed) *History of the Second World War: UK medical services*. London: HMSO

Maggs, C.J. (1983) *The Origins of General Nursing*

Manwaring-White, S. (1983) *The Policing Revolution*. Brighton

Marwick, A. (1974) *War and Social Change in the Twentieth Century*

Posen, B.R. (1984) *The Sources of Military Doctrine*

Romanucci-Ross, L., Moerman, D.E. & Tancredi, L.R. (1983) *The Anthropology of Medicine from Culture to Method*. Massachusetts

Rumbold, G. (1986) *Ethics in Nursing Practice*

Salas, E. (1990) *Soldaderas in the Mexican Military*. Texas

Salvage, J. (1985) *The Politics of Nursing*

Scott, L.V. (1993) *Conscription and the Attlee Government*

Shaw, M. (1991) *Post Military Society*. Cambridge

Splane, R. & Splane, V. (1995) *Chief Nursing Officer Positions in National Ministries of Health*. California

Stanhope, H. (1979) *The Soldiers, an anatomy of the British Army*

Summerfield, P. (1989) *Women Workers in the Second World War*

Summers, A. (1988) *Angels and Citizens*

Taylor, C. (ed) (1970) *In Horizontal Orbit: hospitals and the cult of efficiency*. New York

Titmuss, R. (1958) *Essays on the Welfare State*

Vagts, A. (1967) *A History of Militarism*. New York

Van Doon, J. (ed) (1968) *Armed Forces and Society*. Netherlands

Walby, S. (1986) *Patriarchy at Work*. Minnesota

Walby, S. & Greenwell, J. (1994) *Medicine and the Nursing Professions in a Changing Health Service*

White, R. (1985) *The Effects of the National Health Service on the Nursing Profession*. Kings Fund

Wilkinson, R. (ed) (1969) *Governing Elites, studies in military training and selection*. See in particular 'Correli Barnett, the education of military elite' and 'Otley's study of public schools'

Younghusband, E. (1978) *Social Work in Britain 1950-1975*

Articles

Baly, M. (1996) 'A History of the RCN History Society'. *International History of Nursing Journal*, vol.3

Bourke, J. (1994) 'Housewifery in working class England 1860-1914'. *Past and Present*, 143, 182

Glyn, A. & Sutcliffe, B. (1971) 'The collapse of UK profits'. *New Left Review*, March/April

Hicks, C. (1982) 'Racism in nursing'. *Nursing Times*, 5th May

Kushner, T. (1985) 'An alien occupation'. *Second Chance*

Moores, B. (1971) 'Patterns of nurse wastage'. *International Nursing Studies*, vol.8

Webster, C. (1985) 'The nursing crisis of the early National Health Service'. *Bulletin of the History of Nursing Group*, vol.7

Index

A

American nursing system 125
Area Nurse Training Committees 59, 63
Army Council 30
Association of Hospital Matrons 28, 40, 55, 66, 120, 128, 138
Athlone Interim Report 25, 36
Auxiliary Territorial Service 30, 38

B

Bedford Fenwick, Ethel 19
Bevan, Aneurin 62, 64, 74, 75, 118, 124
Bradbeer Committee & Report 100, 102
Briggs Committee & Report 94, 125, 174, 187, 198, 199, 211, 213, 217, 218
Briggs, Asa 69, 174
British Hospitals Association 65
British Red Cross 28, 31, 38
Brook, Iris 134
Butler Education Reforms 201

C

Cadet Schemes 33, 34, 39, 45, 92, 93, 214
Campaign for Nuclear Disarmament 173
Castle, Barbara 192
Central Health Services Council 120
Civil Nursing Reserve 28, 34, 48
Cockayne, Elizabeth 55, 56, 120
Cohen Report 54, 56, 60, 62, 64, 67, 68
Colonial Office 36, 48, 119
Commonwealth Immigration Act 1968 170
Commonwealth Nurses 41, 42
Confederation of Health Service Employees 22, 120, 126, 134, 135, 136, 137, 166, 182, 183, 185, 189, 192, 193, 212, 214, 217
Conscientious Objectors 19, 20
Conscription 14, 15, 16, 38, 47
Crossman, Richard 126, 185, 187, 190

D

Department of Industrial Administration 91
District Nurses 28, 36, 102, 128
Douglas de Cent, Colonel 162, 189

E

Ely Hospital 185
Emergency Hospital Scheme 25
Equal Pay Act 170

F

Feminist Theory 11, 12

G

General Nursing Council 20, 21, 28, 31, 36, 37, 53, 54, 55, 56, 57, 60, 62, 63, 64, 65, 67, 68, 69, 75, 76, 77, 79, 94, 122, 127, 128, 137, 149, 214, 218, 224, 225
General Nursing Council One Year Registration Courses 76, 77
Godber, George 129, 174
Goddard Report 100
Goodall, Frances 131, 132, 133, 136
Guilleband Report 99

H

Hall, Catherine 179, 189
Halsbury Report 192
Headmasters Association 93
Home Office 76, 89, 122, 161, 163, 167
Horder (Lord) 35, 44, 66
Horder Reports 44, 67, 139, 224
Hospital & Welfare Services Union 120
Hospital Management Committees 101, 179
Hospital Plan 1962 100

I

Industrial Nurses 33
International Council of Nurses 66
International Labour Conference 1949 171

J

Joint Board of Clinical Studies 64, 124
Jones, Katherine 39, 42, 48, 49, 226
Joseph, Keith 191, 192

M

Matriarchal Discipline 200
Mayston Report 125
Mental Health Act 1959 123
Mental Hospital and Institutional Workers Union 119
Militarisation 9, 10, 12, 14, 15, 16, 26, 38, 39, 40, 41, 42, 43, 44, 48, 60, 161, 167, 169, 174, 223, 224, 226
Militarism 9, 12, 13, 14, 15, 16, 17, 18, 19, 22, 43, 47, 49, 173, 194, 199, 204, 208
Military Discipline 43, 100, 204, 209
Ministry of Health 20, 21, 25, 26, 27, 28, 29, 31, 32, 34, 36, 37, 39, 48, 49, 53, 54, 55, 56, 57, 64, 73, 75, 76, 78, 79, 81, 82, 84, 86, 91, 92, 102, 104, 107, 119, 120, 123, 124, 129, 135, 136, 161, 218
Ministry of Labour 21, 32, 36, 48, 54, 56, 57, 73, 75, 77, 81, 84, 89, 91, 127, 130, 131, 184, 214

N

National Association of Local Government Officers 22

National Health Service 10, 11, 49, 53, 54, 57, 63, 73, 74, 78, 87, 90, 99, 100, 101, 103, 108, 109, 118, 119, 120, 122, 123, 124, 128, 129, 135, 136, 154, 160, 170, 171, 177, 179, 180, 181, 192, 201, 223
National Prices and Incomes Board 177
National Union of Public Employees 22, 179, 217
Nightingale 10, 11, 17, 18, 19, 21, 31, 39, 42, 109, 132, 133, 136, 139, 179, 193, 204, 218, 225, 226
Nuffield Hospitals Trust 91, 141, 142
Nurses Act 1943 35, 37
Nurses Act 1949 55, 63, 80, 124

O

Order of St John of Jerusalem 28

P

Pay Pause 1962 161, 177, 180, 182, 184
Platt Report 67, 68
Plowden Report 191
Police Act 1965 173
Police Federation 165, 166
Powell, Enoch 102, 180
Prices and Incomes Policy 104, 188
Prison Officers Union 161
Project 2000 187

Q

Queen Alexandra's Imperial Military Nursing Service 118

R

Racism & racial attitudes 15, 43, 88, 90, 170, 171, 225
Raise the Roof Campaign 104, 162, 188, 189, 192, 193
Raven, Kathleen 64, 101, 120, 121, 124, 211
RCN 136
Regional Health Boards 101, 179
Representation of the Peoples Act 1918 20
Revans (Professor) 11, 210, 215, 216
Royal Army Medical Corps 19, 22, 30, 32
Royal British Nurses Association 19
Royal College of Nursing 17, 21, 44, 55, 56, 57, 63, 65, 66, 67, 80, 101, 102, 104, 118, 119, 120, 122, 127, 128, 131-139, 149, 150-153, 159, 161, 162, 172, 174, 179, 182, 183, 184, 185, 187, 188, 189, 191-193, 194, 205, 224
Royal Medico-Psychological Association 76
Royal Society of Medicine 27
Rushcliffe pay scales 36, 47, 48

S

Salmon Committee 101, 102
Salmon Report & Reforms 83, 100, 103, 104, 105, 125
Salmon, Brian 21, 102, 104, 107, 109, 125
Spanish Civil War 27
Standing Nursing Advisory Committee 64, 103, 120

T

Trades Dispute Act 1906 159
Trenchard (Lord) 165

Trueta (Professor) 27

V

Voluntary Aid Detachment Council 29, 30, 38
Voluntary Aid Detachment Nurses 20, 28, 29, 30, 31, 32, 75

W

War Office 17, 21, 30, 34, 76, 77
Ward, Irene 191
Westmacott, Doris 135, 217
Whitley Council 106, 107, 138, 177, 179, 182, 184, 188, 189, 190, 191, 193
Wilkinson, Louisa 118
Wood Report 53, 55, 56, 57, 59, 60, 62, 64, 66, 122, 124, 197, 213, 224
World Health Organisation 122, 125